THE NURSE'S
SURVIVAL GUIDE

Brenda Goodner, RN, MSN, CS
Linda Skidmore-Roth, RN, MSN

SKIDMORE-ROTH PUBLISHING, INC.

Cover design: Robert Pawlak
Typesetting: Business Support Center
Second edition

Notice: The author(s) and the publisher of this volume have taken care to make certain that all information is correct and compatible with the standards generally accepted at the time of publication.

Goodner, Brenda, 1943-
   The nurse's survival guide/Brenda Goodner, Linda Skidmore-Roth. p. cm.

ISBN 0-944132-75-8
   1. Nursing-Handbooks, manuals, etc. I. Skidmore-Roth, Linda. II. Title
   [DNLM: 1. Nursing Assessment-handbooks. 2. Nursing Process-handbooks.
3. Patient Care Planning-handbooks.
WY 39 G653n]
RT51.G66 1992
610.73-dc19
DNLM/DLC
for Library of Congress 89-5990 CIP
Skidmore-Roth Publishing, Inc.
1001 Wall Street
El Paso, Texas 79915
915-774-0617, 800-825-3150

TABLE OF CONTENTS

INTRODUCTION

ASSESSMENT

CLINICAL VALUES AND STANDARDS

DRUG ADMINISTRATION

CLINICAL SKILLS

NURSING CARE PLANNING

PROFESSIONAL NETWORK

CLINICAL REFERRALS

INTRODUCTION

INTRODUCTION

Table of Contents

HOW TO USE THIS BOOK

The second edition of The Nurse's Survival Guide has been revised and completely updated with suggestions from our readers. New to this edition are assessments for peripheral pulses, cranial nerves, height and weight chart, mini-mental status, Beck's depression inventory, Katz index of activities of daily living, and the Holmes-Rahe social adjustment scale.

This is not just another spector manual in nursing written by uninvolved nurses. This is a book that you can really use, especially when confronted with unfamiliar assignments. This book is about survival--survival in a profession complex with procedures, medications, and responsibilities.

This book is about accountability. By having information readily available, it is hoped that the nurse and the nursing student will increase their accountability in situations where they would otherwise feel uncomfortable. Accountability is the hallmark of nursing care, and nurses are constantly being called upon to fulfill the demands that accountability affords.

I had been teaching a couple of years when a friend who was a director of nurses at a small hospital called and asked me to work during the summer. As always, I needed both the money and the opportunity to hone my clinical skills.

Clinical skills!

Panic flashed through my gut.   IVs.   Codes. Pediatrics!

I had just regained my confidence when my friend stated, "You won't have any trouble. The doctor you will be working with is real nice. He's a cardiologist."

Another flash of panic! ECG skips, monitors, lidocaine drips--does lidocaine mix with D5W or normal saline?

Needless to say, I took the job and showed up with about a dozen of my favorite nursing books--one on ECGs, one on medications, a care plan book, an assessment guide, and a good emergency room book. I thought if I get into a real bind, I'll just look it up. Just a simple matter of survival.

Over the summer, I kept thinking how handy it would be to have all of this information in one book, instead of carrying around a dozen books, each having a few pieces of essential information. I survived the summer, and so did the idea of a book loaded with essential nursing information.

This book is not intended to replace a nursing textbook. Instead, it will complement textbooks as an easy-to-grab handbook. This book presents information that a nurse or nursing student knows, but does not memorize and may need to be refreshed.

It is a handbook loaded with guidelines, assessment forms, and charts of information. This book is not intended to offer extensive rationale. When you do not understand the rational, then it is time to research the subject in a comprehensive textbook on the subject.

THE MARK OF A PROFESSIONAL NURSE

The basic requirements of a profession are:

- Educational requirements;
- Unique knowledge and skills based upon theory;
- Service to society;
- Autonomy in decision-making and practice;
- A code of ethics for practice; and
- Some degree of status within the role.

These requirements are inherent in the foundation of professional nursing. The profession of compassionate caring that Florence Nightingale embraced for nursing is the interpersonal expertise unique to each nurse. These interpersonal skills are intimately interwined with the professional skills.

Interpersonal skills encompass all the human actions that respect the body, mind and spirit of another person. It is looking at the patient with kindness, listening with empathy and responding with compassion. A professional nurse offers much more than technical skills, although more and more technical skills are required. It is the interpersonal skills that exhibit caring, confidentiality and positive regard for the patient in a holistic vision that are most valued in the professional nurse.

What do patients want in a nurse? This question was asked of several patients in the process of writing this book. What they want is empathy, sensitivity, experience (skills), caring and a sense of confidence, in that order. What they do not want is a nurse who is insensitive, in a hurry, with an air of power. Patients tend to feel very uncomfortable around nurses who seem unsure of what they are doing.

The quality of caring is not measured by time. The wink of an eye, the flash of a smile, the tenderness of a touch does not require extra time--it demonstrates nursing care.

It is impossible to label the characteristic that makes a nurse professional. That essential quality is elusive, perhaps indescribable. But, when you meet a nurse that has it, you know.

STANDARDS OF CLINICAL NURSING PRACTICE

The American Nurses Association sets a standard for nursing that focuses on practice. When nursing care is measured, accountability is also measured on how these standards are concurrently utilized. The ANA Standards of Clinical Nursing Practice are used for measuring accountability in nursing.

The first standards were published in 1973. In 1989, a task force began revising these standards, and these new standards were published in 1991. The major change is the new emphasis on clinical nursing practice. The standards now address the full scope of practice and is divided into two parts: Standards of Care and Standards of Professional Performance.

Standards of Care

- Assessment
- Diagnosis
- Outcome identification
- Planning

- Implementation
- Evaluation
- Standards of professional performance
- Quality of care
- Performance appraisal
- Education
- Collegiality
- Ethics
- Collaboration
- Research
- Resource utilization

"Standards of Care" describe a competent level of nursing care as demonstrated by the nursing process, involving assessment, diagnosis, outcome identification, planning, implementation, and evaluation. The nursing process encompasses all significant actions taken by nurses in providing care to all clients, and forms the foundation of clinical decision making. Additional nursing responsibilities for all clients (such as providing culturally and ethnically relevant care, maintaining a safe environment, educating clients about their illness, treatment, health promotion or self-care activities, and planning for continuity of care) are explained within these standards. Therefore, "Standards of Care" delineate care that is provided to all clients of nursing services.

STANDARDS OF PROFESSIONAL PERFORMANCE

"Standards of Professional Performance" describe a competent level of behavior in the professional role including activities related to quality of care, performance appraisal, education, collegiality, ethics, collaboration, research, and resource utilization. All nurses are expected to engage in professional role activities appropriate to their education, position, and practice setting. While this is an assumption of all of the "Standards of Professional Performance", the scope of nursing involvement in some professional roles is particularly dependent upon the nurse's education, position, and practice environment. Therefore, some standards or measurement criteria identify a broad range of activities that may demonstrate compliance with the standards.

STANDARDS OF CARE

Standard I. Assessment

The Nurse collects Client Health Data.

Measurement criteria

1. The priority of data collection is determined by the client's immediate condition or needs.

2. Pertinent data are collected using appropriate assessment techniques.

3. Data collection involves the client, significant others, and health care providers when appropriate.

4. The data collection process is systematic and ongoing.

5. Relevant data are documented in a retrievable form.

Standard II. Diagnosis

The nurse analyzes the assessment data in determining diagnoses.

Measurement Criteria

1. Diagnoses are derived from the assessment data.
2. Diagnoses are validated with the client, significant others, and health care providers, when possible.
3. Diagnoses are documented in a manner that facilitates the determination of unexpected outcomes and plan of care.

Standard III. Outcome Identification

The nurse identifies expected outcomes individualized to the client.

Measurement Criteria

1. Outcomes are derived from the diagnoses.
2. Outcomes are documented as measurable goals.
3. Outcomes are mutually formulated with the client and health care providers, when possible.
4. Outcomes are realistic in relation to the client's present and potential capabilities.
5. Outcomes are attainable in relation to resources available to the client.
6. Outcomes include a time estimate for attainment.
7. Outcomes provide direction for continuity of care.

Standard IV. Planning

The nurse develops a plan of care that prescribes interventions to attain expected outcomes.

Measurement Criteria

1. The plan is individualized to the client's condition or needs.
2. The plan is developed with the client, significant others, and health care providers, when appropriate.
3. The plan reflects current nursing practice.
4. The plan is documented.
5. The plan provides for continuity of care.

Standard V. Implementation

The nurse implements the interventions identified in the plan of care.

Measurement Criteria

1. Interventions are consistent with the established plan of care.
2. Interventions are implemented in a safe and appropriate manner.
3. Interventions are documented.

Standard VI. Evaluation

The nurse evaluates the client's progress toward attainment of outcomes.

Measurement Criteria

1. Evaluation is systematic and ongoing.

2. The client's responses to interventions are documented.

3. The effectiveness of interventions is evaluated in relation to outcomes.

4. Ongoing assessment data are used to revise diagnoses, outcomes, and the plan of care, as needed.

5. Revisions in diagnoses, outcomes, and the plan of care are documented

6. The client, significant others, and health care providers are involved in the evaluation process, when appropriate.

STANDARDS OF PROFESSIONAL PERFORMANCE

Standard I. Quality of Care

The nurse systematically evaluates the quality and effectiveness of nursing practice.

Measurement Criteria

1. The nurse participates in quality of care activities as appropriate to the individual's position, education, and practice environment. Such activities may include:

   · Identification of aspects of care important for quality monitoring.

   · Identification of indicators used to monitor quality and effectiveness of nursing care.

   · Collection of data to monitor quality and effectiveness of nursing care.

- Analysis of quality data to identify opportunities for improving care.
- Formulation of recommendations to improve nursing practice or client outcomes.
- Implementation of activities to enhance the quality of nursing practice.
- Participation on interdisciplinary teams that evaluate clinical practice or health services.
- Development of policies and procedures to improve quality of care.

2. The nurse uses the results of quality of care activities to initiate changes in practice.
3. The nurse uses the results of quality of care activities to initiate changes throughout the health care delivery system, as appropriate.

Standard II. Performance Appraisal

The nurse evaluates his/her own nursing practice in relation to professional practice standards and relevant statutes and regulations.

Measurement Criteria

1. The nurse engages in performance appraisal on a regular basis, identifying areas of strength as well as areas for professional/practice development.
2. The nurse seeks constructive feedback regarding his/her own practice.

3. The nurse takes action to achieve goals identified during performance appraisal.
4. The nurse participates in peer review as appropriate.

Standard III. Education

The nurse acquires and maintains current knowledge in nursing practice.

Measurement Criteria

1. The nurse participates in ongoing educational activities related to clinical knowledge and professional issues.
2. The nurse seeks experiences to maintain clinical skills.
3. The nurse seeks knowledge and skill appropriate to the practice setting.

Standard IV. Collegiality

The nurse contributes to the professional development of peers, colleagues, and others.

Measurement Criteria

1. The nurse shares knowledge and skill with colleagues and others.
2. The nurse provides peers with constructive feedback regarding their practice.
3. The nurse contributes to an environment that is conducive to clinical education of nursing students, as appropriate.

Standard V. Ethics

The nurse's decisions and actions on behalf of clients are determined in an ethical manner.

Measurement Criteria

1. The nurse's practice is guided by the Code for Nurses.
2. The nurse maintains client confidentiality.
3. The nurse acts as a client advocate.
4. The nurse delivers care in a nonjudgmental and nondiscriminatory manner that is sensitive to client diversity.
5. The nurse delivers in a manner that preserves/protects client autonomy, dignity, and rights.
6. The nurse seeks available resources to help formulate ethical decisions.

Standard VI. Collaboration

The nurse collaborates with the client, significant others, and health care providers in providing client care.

Measurement Criteria

1. The nurse communicates with the client, significant others, and health care providers regarding client care and nursing's role in the provision of care.
2. The nurse consults with health care providers for client care, as needed.
3. The nurse makes referrals, including provisions for continuity of care, as needed.

Standard VII. Research

The nurse uses research findings in practice.

Measurement Criteria

1. The nurse uses interventions substantiated by research as appropriate to the individual's position, education, and practice environment.

2. The nurse participates in research activities as appropriate to the individual's position, education, and practice environment. Such activities may include:

   · Identification of clinical problems suitable for nursing research.

   · Participation in data collection.

   · Participation in a unit, organization, or community research committee or program.

   · Sharing of research activities with others.

   · Conducting research.

   · Critiquing research for application to practice.

   · Using research findings in the development of policies, procedures, and guidelines for client care.

Standard VIII. Resource Utilization

The nurse considers factors related to safety, effectiveness, and cost in planning and delivering client care.

Measurement Criteria.

1. The nurse evaluates factors related to safety, effectiveness, and cost when two or more practice options would result in the same expected client outcome.

2. The nurse assigns tasks or delegates care based on the needs of the client and the knowledge and skill of the provider selected.

3. The nurse assists the client and significant others in identifying and securing appropriate services available to address health-related needs.

Printed with permission of the American Nurses Association from the ANA's Standards of Nursing Practice, 1991.

ASSESSMENT

ASSESSMENT

Table of Contents

THE HEAD-TO-TOE SYSTEMS ASSESSMENT

GENERAL STATUS

Age
Sex
Race
General health status/personal appearance
Physical motor activity
General nutritional status
Previously diagnosed disease
Height/weight
Emotional status/affect
Verbal response/degree of cooperation

VITAL SIGNS

Temperature
Pulse
    Carotid
    Apical
    Brachial
    Radial
    Femoral
    Popliteal
    Posterior tibialis
    Dorsalis pedis
Respirations
    Rate
    Depth
    Regularity
    Mouth/nasal

Blood Pressure
  Sitting
  Lying
  Standing
  Right arm/left arm

RESPIRATORY SYSTEM

Breath Sounds
  Normal
  Adventitious
Cough
  Productive
  Non-productive
Dyspnea
Hemoptysis
Orthopnea
Paroxysmal nocturnal dyspnea
Breath odor
  Fruity
  Fetid
  Alcohol
  Ammonia
Chest
  Symmetry
  Pain
Sinus
  Pain
  Drainage
  Infections
Nose
  Epistaxis

Postnasal drip
Deviated septum

CARDIOVASCULAR SYSTEM

Cardiac Patterns
Rate
Rhythm
PMI (point of maximum impulse)
Thrills
Murmurs
ECG strip (date of last ECG)
Palpitations
Pacemaker
Vessels
Carotid
Jugular
Strength of pulses
Symmetry of pulses
Bruits
Capillary refill
Varicosities
Thrombophlebitis
Lymph nodes
Enlargement
Shape
Mobility
Tenderness

INTEGUMENTARY SYSTEM

Skin color
Pink/natural

Pale
Erythema
Jaundice
Cyanotic
Mottled
Blanched
Vascularity
  Bruises
  Bleeding
  Ecchymosis
  Petechiae
Edema
  +1--Slight pitting, normal contour
  +2--Deeper, contours still present
  +3--Deep pittting, puffy appearance
  +4--Deep pitting, frankly swollen
Temperature
Turgor
Texture
  Scars
  Dryness
  Pruritis
Lesions, rash
  Type
  Size
  Color
  Shape
  Distribution
Masses
  Size
  Shape

Location
Mobility
Tenderness
Nails
Texture
Color
Lines
Hair
Distribution
Color
Texture

NEUROLOGICAL SYSTEM

Level of Consciousness
Alert, oriented
Lethargic
Obtunded
Stuporous
Semicomatose
Comatose
Head
Pain
Lesions
Edema
Bumps
Face
Symmetry
Expression
Color
Eyes
Acuity

Glasses
Contacts
Prosthesis
Amblyopia
Photophobia
Diplopia
Strabismus
Nystagmus
Pain
Cataracts
Glaucoma
Pruritis
Redness
Discharge
Ptosis
Conjunctiva
Sclera
Vascularity
Pupils
Size
Shape
PERRLA
Neck
Symmetry
ROM
Pain
Stiffness
Extremities
Tingling
Edema
Stiffness

Pain
Reflexes
   Deep tendon reflexes
   Biceps
   Triceps
   Patellar
   Achilles tendon
Superficial reflexes
   Pharyngeal
   Abdominal
   Plantar
Grading reflexes
   O--No Response
   1+--Diminished
   2+--Normal
   3+--Brisk
   4+--Hyperactive

Ears
   Loss of hearing/hearing aid
   Infections
   Tinnitus
   Vertigo
   Wax deposits
   History of seizures

GASTROINTESTINAL SYSTEM

Appetite
Pain
Indigestion
Nausea/vomiting

Mouth/throat
  Color
  Odor
  Pain
  Speech/hoarseness
  Swallowing
  Chewing
  Taste
  Ulcerations
  Lesions
  Teeth/dentures/gums
  Bleeding
  Gag reflex
Abdomen
  Size/contour
  Symmetry
  Muscle tone/adipose
Scars/Striae
  Fluid/ascites
Distention/Rigidity
  Bowel sounds RUQ, RLQ, LUQ, LLQ
    Hypoactive
    Hyeractive
Pain/Guarding
Liver Border/Splenic Dullness
Rectum
  Hemorrhoids
  Excoriation/lesions
  Rash/itching
  Abcess
  Pilonidal cysts
  Burning/pain

Bowel Elimination
   Normal pattern
   Diarrhea
   Constipation
   Flatus
   Use of laxatives

RENAL SYSTEM

Urinary Output
   Amount
   Color
   Odor
   Frequency
   Urgency
   Hesitancy
   Burning/Pain
   Dribbling
   Hematuria
   Nocturia
   Oliguria
   Polyuria
Bladder Distention
Flank Pain
Stress Incontinence
Daily Fluid Intake
   Water
   Alcohol
   Soft drinks
   Caffeine

MUSCULOSKELETAL SYSTEM

Level of Activity
Extremities
  Size/shape
  Symmetry
  Color
  Warmth
  ROM
  Scars
  Bruises
  Rash
  Ulcerations
  Numbness
  Tingling
  Edema
  Prosthesis
  Fracture
  Infection/bone
  Intermittent Claudication
Joints
  ROM
  Deformities
  Stiffness
  Edema
  Pain/tenderness
Muscles
  Conditioning/tone
  Spasms
  Tremors
  Weakness

Back
  Pain
  Spinal abnormalities
  Kyphosis
  Scoliosis

REPRODUCTIVE SYSTEM

Male
  Penis
      Discharge
      Ulceration
      Prepuce
      Pain
  Scrotum
      Edema
      Nodules
      Ulceration
      Tenderness
  Testes
      Edema
      Masses
  Prostate
      Masses
      Tenderness
 Female
    Discharge
    Edema
    Ulceration
    Nodules
    Masses
    Pain/tenderness

Onset of LMP
Menstrual abnormalities
History of venereal disease
Last pap smear
Method of birth control
Breasts
   Discharge
   Contour
   Symmetry
   Inflammation
   Scars
   Masses
      Location
      Size
      Mobility
      Pain/tenderness
      Dimpling
      Nipple discharge
      Nipple inversion
      Ulcerations
      Last breast exam
   Axillae
      Nodes
      Enlargement
      Tenderness
      Rash

ENDOCRINE SYSTEM

General growth and development
Previous diagnosis
Presence of secondary sex characteristics

Exophthalmos
Goiter
Hormone therapy
Polydipsia
Polyuria
Polyphagia
Postural hypotension

CENTRAL NERVOUS SYSTEM

Previous diagnosis
Anxiety
Loss of Consciousness (history)
Behavior Changes
Mood Swings
Nervousness
Seizures
Sensory Problems
Cognitive Ability
Memory
    Recent
    Present
    Remote
Psychomotor
    Ataxia
    Paralysis
    Tremor
    Spasm

SEQUENCE OF PHYSICAL EXAMINATION

1. Wash hands
2. Assemble equipment
3. Approach patient with a sincere, caring attitude
4. Explain assessment procedure to patient
5. Measure height, weight, vital signs
6. Take history
7. Perform system assessment
8. Check facial expression or unusual movements
9. Inspect eyes for PERRLA
10. Check corneal blink reflex
11. Inspect ears
12. Check mouth and gag reflex
13. Check ROM of neck
14. Palpate neck, check lymph nodes
15. Palpate thyroid
16. Palpate carotid and radial pulses
17. Inspect chest symmetry
18. Determine pattern of respiration
19. Inspect spine
20. Auscultate posterior lung fields
21. Inspect anterior chest
22. Inspect breasts and axilla
23. Percuss and auscultate anterior lung fields
24. Inspect hands and arms
25. Check arm, elbow and wrist ROM
26. Auscultate heart sounds
27. Ask patient to assume supine postition
28. Inspect and palpate abdomen and flanks

29. Auscultate bowel sounds, bruits
30. Percuss liver
31. Inspect inguinal area
32. Palpate, auscultate femoral arteries
33. Check legs for ROM and muscular strength
34. Palpate popliteal and pedal pulses
35. Inspect and palpate genitalia
36. Check deep tendon reflexes and Babinski's sign

BREATH SOUNDS

Breath sounds are the sounds heard as air moves through the tracheobronchoaveolar system during inspiration and expiration. It is important to differentiate between normal and abnormal (adventitious) breath sounds when assessing a patient.

NORMAL BREATH SOUNDS

BREATH SOUND	INTENSITY/ RATIO	NORMAL	ABNORMAL
Vesicular	Soft, breezy; 3-1 ratio, higher	Heard over lung on periphery at 2nd ICS	When not heard and over trachea
Bronchial	High, loud; 2-3 ratio	Midline over trachea or main bronchus	Over lung fields, especially peripheral, indicates atelectasis
Broncho-vesicular	Moderate; 1-1 ratio	Heard over upper airways at 2nd ICS bilaterally	Decreased over periphery, may indicate pneumonia

ADVENTITIOUS BREATH SOUNDS

Crackles	Soft, crackling, bubbling; more obvious on inspiration	Widespread over peripheral fields and lung bases	Pneumonia, pulmonary edema, early CHF
Rhonchi	Gurgling, course, rattling, musical. More obvious on expiration	Bronchi, trachea	Bronchitis, emphysema, pneumonia CHF

BREATH SOUND	INTENSITY/ RATIO	NORMAL	ABNORMAL
Wheezes	High-pitched whistling, creaking, accentuated during expiration	All lung fields, airways	Asthma, COPD
Pleural friction rub	Grating on inspiration and expiration. Inspiration accentuated	Anterior, peripheral fields	TB, lung cancer, inflammation of pleural surfaces

RESPIRATORY PATTERNS

In assessing the rate, rhythm, and depth of respirations, always count for one minute. It is best to observe the patient at rest without his awareness of your counting. If he is aware that you are counting, this may alter his pattern of respiration.

DESCRIP- TION	RATE	RHYTHM AND DEPTH	POSSIBLE ETIOLOGY
Eupnea	Normal: Neonate:30-50 Child age 2: 20-30; Child age 10: 14-22; Adult and Adolescent: 12-20	Regular with occasional deep breaths	Absence of disease process
Bradypnea	Slower than normal rate	Regular with occasional deep breaths	Normal when sleeping, narcotics, alcohol, respiratory decompensa-

DESCRIP-TION	RATE	RHYTHM AND DEPTH	POSSIBLE ETIOLOGY
			tion, metabolic disorders
Tachypnea	Faster than normal rate	Steady and shallow	Fever, over-activity
Apnea	Absence of respiration	None	Periodic when sleeping
Hyperpnea	Normal	Deeper than normal, faster than normal	Assess activity, may not be abnormal if activity strenuous
Cheyne-Stokes respiration	Faster for first few seconds, then slower; will last 30 to 120 second	Deeper than normal with periods of shallow respir-ation and apnea varying from 20-60 seconds	Critically ill
Kussmaul respiration	20 breaths faster per minute	Deep, labored breaths	Renal failure, metabolic acidosis

LANDMARKS FOR BREATH
SOUNDS ASSESSMENT

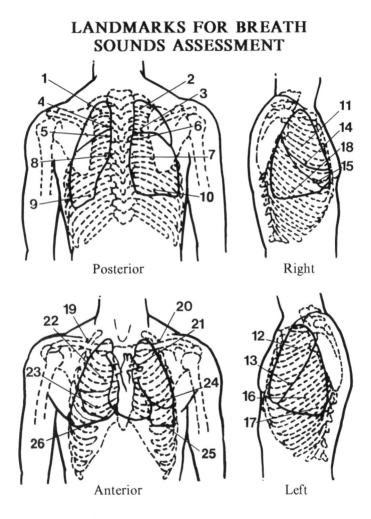

Posterior   Right

Anterior   Left

Place stethoscope at the landmarks designated.   The
stethoscope should be moved in the designated sequence.

ASSESSING HEART SOUNDS

SOUND	OCCURS	LOCATION	MIMICS
S₁	Closure of atrioventricular valves (mitral and tricuspid). Systole begins.	Entire precordium. Best at apex.	LUB-dub
S₂	Closure of semi-lunar valves (aortic and pulmonic). Diastole begins.	Entire precordium. Best at base.	lub-DUB
S₃	First phase of rapid ventricular filling.	Apex with bell.	Ken-TUC-ky
S₄	Second phase of ventricular filling with forceful atrial ejection.	Apex with bell.	TEN-nes-see

Landmarks for heart sound assessment

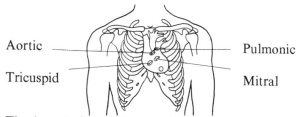

Aortic   Pulmonic

Tricuspid   Mitral

The heart's four valves and their sound transmission routes are located on this diagram. The circled letters identify auscultation sites.

ASSESSMENT OF PERIPHERAL PULSES

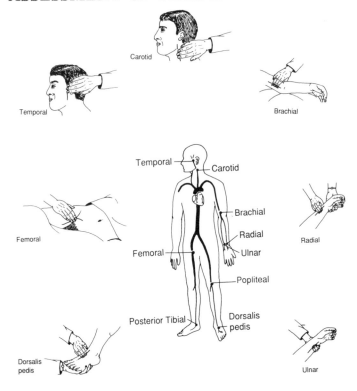

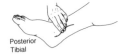

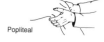

ASSESSMENT OF THE CRANIAL NERVES

NERVE	FUNCTION	ASSESSMENT
I Olfactory	Sense of smell	With patient's eyes closed occlude one nostril at a time. Using a stimulus such as coffee, chocolate, or vanilla, ask the patient to identify the smell.
II Optic	Visual	(1) Test visual acuity with Snellen chart. (2) Inspect optic fundi with opthalmoscope to assess optic disc and retinal vessels. (3) Inspect retina for lesions. (4) Face patient, 2-3 feet away, asking patient to cover one eye. Move small white object slowly from periphery to center until the patient sees it. Note the expanse of the visual field.

NERVE	FUNCTION	ASSESSMENT
III Oculomotor	Eye movement	Assess pupil size and reaction to light. Check for drooping. To assess the six cardinal fields of gaze, ask the patient to follow your finger as you move it horizontally left and right, then vertically. Assess for failure to move or involuntary movements.
IV Trochlear	Eye movement	Same as CN III
V Trigeminal	Facial and scalp movement, chewing	(1) Assess jaw opening by feeling the masseter muscle and chewing temporalis as patient bites down. (2) Observe response to lightly touching each cornea with a small wisp of sterile cotton.
VI Abducens	Turning eyes outward	Same as CN III and IV
VII Facial	Controls facial muscles, sense of taste	1. Ask patient to smile, frown, wrinkle forehead,

NERVE	FUNCTION	ASSESSMENT
		squeeze eyes shut while checking for symmetry. 2. Place sugar and salt on each side of tongue to test for taste.
VIII Acoustic	Hearing, sense of balance	Whisper to test sense of hearing. Compare air and bone conduction.
IX Glosso-pharyngeal	Sense of taste, gag reflex and swallowing	Same as for VII Same as for X
X Vagus	Swallowing, gag reflex, vocal sounds	Touch back of tongue with tongue blade, ask patient to say "ah". Observe for symmetry and upward movement of palate. Observe for hoarseness. Assess ability to swallow water.
XI Spinal Accessory	Head and shoulder movements	Assess strength and size of sternocleidomastoid and trapezius muscle.
XII Hypo-glossal	Tongue movements	Assess size and movement of tongue. Assess strength with

NERVE	FUNCTION	ASSESSMENT
		with patient pushing tongue against cheek while applying resistance with index finger. Note any deviations in vocal sounds.

PAIN ASSESSMENT

P - Point of origin.

Where did it start? (Point with index finger.)
When did it start?
What were you doing at the time it started?
Where does it spread?

A - Alleviating/aggravating factors.

What makes it better?
What makes it worse?
Has this pain occurred before? If so, what happened?
Do you take pain medication?
What is the level of anxiety?

I - Intensity.

How does it rate on a scale of 1 to 5 with 1 for mild
discomfort and 5 for intolerable pain?

N - Nature of the pain.

Describe the pain: discomfort, distress, burning,
constricting, gnawing, cramping, crushing.

NUTRITIONAL ASSESSMENT

Diet dramatically affects a person's state of health. To assess a patient's nutritional status, first record the typical 24-hour intake, then assess eating habits on a weekly basis. After completing the assessment, you can evaluate the adequacy of the diet according to the guidelines established by the basic four food groups.

Nutritional Assessment Form

Name
Age
Date
Sex
Marital status
Occupation
Height and weight
Recent weight loss
Recent weight gain
Medical diagnosis
Food restrictions (medical or religious)
Ethnic and economic background
Problems with eating (dentures, chewing, swallowing)
Food allergies
Food preferences
Daily nutritional supplements
Patient complaints (weakness, indigestion, skin problems)
Elimination habits
Use of laxatives

24-HOUR FOOD INTAKE FORM

TIME	FOOD	*PREPARATION	AMOUNT	FOOD GROUP

* Home-cooked or store pre-prepared

Evaluation of Nutritional Assessment

Adequate intake of vitamin A   YES   NO

Adequate intake of vitamin C

Adequate intake of protein

Adequate intake of calcium

Adequate intake of calories

Adequate intake of complex carbohydrates

THE BASIC FOUR FOOD GROUPS GUIDE

FOOD GROUP	SERVINGS REQUIRED PER DAY	NUTRIENTS SUPPLIED
Dairy products	Adults, 2 cups Children, 4 cups	Protein, calcium vitamins A and D (when fortified)
Fruits and vegetables	4 servings, including at least 1 serving of green or yellow vegetables and 1 serving of citrus fruit	Vitamin A and C; fiber*
Meat, fish, eggs, legumes	2 or more servings	Protein, iron, niacin, thiamin
Bread, cereal, grains	4 or more servings	Thiamin, niacin, complex carbohydrates

*Fiber is not a nutrient, but is essential in dietary intake.

RECOMMENDED DIETARY ALLOWANCES

The following guidelines are designed for the maintenance of good nutrition of practically all healthy people in the U.S.A.

	Age	Weight		Height		Protein
	(years)	(kg)	(lb.)	(cm)	(in.)	(g)
Infants	0.0-0.5	6	13	60	24	13
	0.5-1.0	9	20	71	28	14
Children	1-3	13	29	90	35	16
	4-6	20	44	112	44	24
	7-10	28	62	132	52	28
Males	11-14	45	99	157	62	45
	15-18	66	145	176	69	59
	19-24	72	160	177	70	58
	25-50	79	174	176	70	63
	51+	77	170	173	68	63
Females	11-14	46	101	157	62	46
	15-18	55	120	163	64	44
	19-24	58	128	164	65	46
	25-50	63	138	163	64	50
	51+	65	143	160	63	50

Fat-Soluble Vitamins

	Age (years)	Vitamin A (mg)	Vitamin D (mg)	Vitamin E (mg)	Vitamin K (ug)
Infants	0.0-0.5	375	7.5	3	5
	0.5-1.0	375	10	4	10
Children	1-3	400	10	6	15
	4-6	500	10	7	20
	7-10	700	10	7	30
Males	11-14	1000	10	10	45
	15-18	1000	10	10	65
	19-24	1000	10	10	70
	25-50	1000	5	10	80
	51+	1000	5	10	80
Females	11-14	800	10	8	45
	15-18	800	10	8	55
	19-24	800	10	8	60
	25-50	800	5	8	65
	51+	800	5	8	65
Pregnant		+800	+10	+10	65
Lactating					
1st 6 months		1300	10	12	65
2nd 6 months		1200	10	11	65

Water-Soluble Vitamins

	Age (years)	Vitamin C (mg)	Thiamin (mg)	Riboflavin (mg)	Niacin (mg)	Vit. B6 (mg)
Infants	0.0-0.5	30	0.3	0.4	5	0.3
	0.5-1.0	35	0.4	0.5	6	0.6
Children	1-3	40	0.7	0.8	9	1.0
	4-6	45	0.9	1.1	12	1.1
	7-10	45	1.0	1.2	13	1.4
Males	11-14	50	1.3	1.5	17	1.7
	15-18	60	1.5	1.8	20	2.0
	19-24	60	1.5	1.7	19	2.0
	25-50	60	1.1	1.3	15	1.6
	51+	60	1.0	1.2	13	1.6
Females	11-14	50	1.1	1.3	15	1.4
	15-18	60	1.1	1.3	15	1.5
	19-24	60	1.1	1.3	15	1.6
	25-50	60	1.1	1.3	15	1.6
	51+	60	1.0	1.2	13	1.6
Pregnant		70	1.5	1.6	17	2.2
Lactating						
1st 6 months		95	1.6	1.8	20	2.2
2nd 6 months		90	1.6	1.7	20	2.1

Water-Soluble Vitamins

	Age (years)	Folate (Ug)	Vitamin B12 (Ug)
Infants	0.0-0.5	25	0.3
	0.5-1.0	35	0.5
Children	1-3	50	0.7
	4-6	75	1.0
	7-10	100	1.4
Males	11-14	150	2.0
	15-18	200	2.0
	19-24	200	2.0
	25-50	200	2.0
	51+	200	2.0

	Age (years)	Folate (Ug)	Vitamin B12 (Ug)
Female	11-14	150	2.0
	15-18	180	2.0
	19-24	180	2.0
	25-50	180	2.0
	51+	180	2.0
Pregnant		400	2.2
Lactating			
1st 6 months		280	2.6
2nd 6 months		260	2.6

MINERALS

	Age (years)	Calcium (mg)	Phosphorus (mg)	Magnesium (mg)	Iron (mg)	Zinc (mg)
Infants	0.0-0.5	400	300	40	6	5
	0.5-1.0	600	500	60	10	5
Children	1-3	800	800	80	10	10
	4-6	800	800	120	10	10
	7-10	800	800	170	10	10
Males	11-14	1200	1200	270	12	15
	15-18	1200	1200	400	12	15
	19-24	1200	1200	350	10	15
	25-50	800	800	350	10	15
	51+	800	800	350	10	15
Females	11-14	1200	1200	280	15	12
	15-15	1200	1200	300	15	12
	19-24	1200	1200	280	15	12
	25-50	800	800	280	15	12
	51+	800	800	280	10	12
Pregnant		1200	1200	300	30	15
Lactating						
1st 6 months		1200	1200	355	15	19
2nd 6 months		1200	1200	340	15	16

Minerals

	Age (years)	Iodine (mg)	Selenium (mg)
Infants	0.0-0.5	40	10
	0.5-1.0	50	15
Children	1-3	70	20
	4-6	90	20
	7-10	120	30
Males	11-14	150	40
	15-18	150	50
	19-24	150	70
	25-50	150	70
	51+	150	70
Females	11-14	150	45
	15-18	150	50
	19-24	150	55
	25-50	150	55
	51+	150	55
Pregnant		175	65
Lactating			
1st 6 mo		200	75
2nd 6 mo		200	75

Food and Nutrition Board, National Academy of Sciences National Research Council Recommended Daily Dietary Allowances; Revised 1989.

WHAT THE NUTRIENTS DO

VITAMIN A

Fat-soluble

RDA: 800-1,000 ug RE

ROLE

Repairs tissue, aids in resistance of infection. Maintains healthy skin, hair, mucous membranes, adequate night vision, bone growth, teeth development, reproduction and RNA synthesis.

SIGNS OF DEFICIENCY

Night blindness, infection of mucous membranes, dry mucous membranes, dry, rough skin, increased susceptibility to infections, sinus infections.

BEST SOURCES

Fish, green and yellow vegetables, dairy products, carrots (raw is best), liver, spinach.

VITAMIN B_1 (Thiamin)

Water-soluble

RDA: 1.0-1.5 mg.

ROLE

Maintains carbohydrate metabolism, energy levels, circulation, digestion, muscle tone, nervous system.

SIGNS OF DEFICIENCY

Beriberi, constipation, fatigue, irritability, nervousness.

SOURCES

Brewer's yeast, eggs, molasses, fish, meat, poultry, nuts.

B_2 (Riboflavin)

Water-soluble

RDA: 1.0-1.5 mg.

ROLE

Maintains RBC and antibody formation, metabolism, cell utilization of oxygen, normal nerve structure, healthy lips, mouth and tongue.

SIGNS OF DEFICIENCY

Cracks in lips, red sore tongue, dizziness, poor digestion.

SOURCES

Eggs, green leafy vegetables, nuts, legumes, organ meats, poultry, whole grains, whole milk.

B_6 (Pyridoxine)

Water-soluble

RDA: 1.4-2.0 mg

ROLE

Maintains antibody function, digestion, DNA and RNA synthesis, hemoglobin production, maintains sodium and potassium balance, nerve function, tryptophane conversion.

SIGNS OF DEFICIENCY

Anemia, hair loss, irritability, weakness, depression.

SOURCES

Meats, liver, whole grains, beans, milk, bananas, prunes.

B_{12} (Cobalamin)

Water-soluble

RDA: 2.0 ug

ROLE

Maintains blood cell formation, appetite, healthy nervous system, iron absorption.

SIGNS OF DEFICIENCY

Fatigue, memory impairment, depression, confusion, nervousness, pernicious anemia, weakness.

SOURCES

Beef, eggs, fish, milk, pork.

FOLIC ACID

Water-soluble

RDA: 180-200 ug

ROLE

Maintains cell growth and reproduction, DNA production, RBC formation, protein metabolism.

SIGNS OF DEFICIENCY

Anemia, digestive problems, insomnia, inflammation of tongue, memory impairment.

SOURCES

Legunes, eggs, green leafy vegetables, milk, liver, seafood, whole grains.

NIACIN

Water-soluble

RDA: 13-19 mg.

ROLE

Aids growth and circulation, reduces cholesterol, maintains metabolism, sex hormone production.

SIGNS OF DEFICIENCY

Loss of appetite, canker sores, depression, fatigue, headaches, nervous disorders, muscular weakness; pellagra which includes symptoms of diarrhea, severe dermatitis, dementia.

SOURCES

Eggs, lean meats, milk, poultry, whole grains, seafood.

VITAMIN C

Water-soluble

RDA: 50-60 mg.

ROLE

Maintains collagen production, bone and tooth formation, healing processes, RBC formation, resistance to infections.

SIGNS OF DEFICIENCY

Anemia, bleeding gums, easily bruised, low resistance to infections, nosebleeds, poor digestion, scurvy.

SOURCES

Orange juice, citrus fruits, broccoli, green peppers, strawberries.

VITAMIN D

Fat-soluble

RDA: 5-10 ug

ROLE

Aids in calcium absorption, bone formation, maintains nervous system, normal blood clotting.

SIGNS OF DEFICIENCY

Insomnia, diarrhea, softening of bones and teeth, rickets, osteomalacia, osteoporosis.

SOURCES

Egg yolk, liver, sunlight, mild, salmon, tuna. Note: As cholecalciferol, 10 ug cholecalciferol equals 400 IU of Vitamin D.

VITAMIN E

Fat-Soluble

RDA: 8-10 IU

ROLE

Maintains muscles and nerves, antioxident, strengthens capillary walls.

SIGNS OF DEFICIENCY

Nervousness, dry, falling hair, muscular weakness. Deficiency is difficult to detect because it is rare.

SOURCES

Butter, eggs, fruit, nuts, vegetables, oil, wheat germ.

VITAMIN K

Fat-soluble

RDA: 45-80 ug.

ROLE

Coagulation of blood (clotting)

SIGNS OF DEFICIENTY

Increased tendency to hemorrhage, nosebleeds.

SOURCES

Green leafy vegetables, oatmeal, liver.

PROTEIN

RDA: 50-60 mg.

ROLE

Builds and maintains all body tissue, builds blood and aids in formation of antibodies to fight infection, supplies food energy after carbohydrates and fats are burned.

SIGNS OF DEFICIENCY

Muscle wasting, decreased resistance to infection, decreased energy levels. In advanced stages, Kwashiorkor.

SOURCES

Complete proteins: meat, fish, poultry, eggs, milk, cheese. Incomplete proteins: peas, beans, bread, cereals, nuts.

CARBOHYDRATES

Recommended intake of carbohydrates: 60-65%.

ROLE

Supplies energy, helps body use other nutrients

SIGNS OF DEFICIENCY

Decreased energy levels, fatigue

SOURCES

Breads, cereals, rice, spaghetti, potatoes, corn, dried fruits, bananas, sugar, jams, honey.

FATS

Recommended intake of fat: 10-30%.

ROLE

Supplies large amount of energy in a small amount of food, supplies essential fatty acids needed for use and storage of fats.

SIGNS OF DEFICIENCY

Muscle wasting because protein is used for energy instead of fat.

SOURCES

Butter, salad oils, fats in meat, especially bacon, milk, eggs, nuts.

CALCIUM

RDA: 800-1200 mg.

ROLE

Maintains bones and teeth, muscle growth, regulates heart beat, assists in blood clotting.

SIGNS OF DEFICIENCY

Rickets, osteoporosis, muscle cramps, increased susceptibility to fractures.

SOURCES

Dairy products, salmon, sardines, nuts, beans.

CHLORIDE

ESI: 1,800-5,000 mg.

ROLE

Maintains acid and alkali levels in blood, digestion, liver function, and waste elimination.

SIGNS OF DEFICIENCY

Rare, possible acid/base disturbance.

SOURCES

Salt, ripe olives, fish, smoked meats.

PHOSPHORUS

RDA: 800 mg.

ROLE

Maintains strong bones and teeth, heart beat regulation, kidney function, an important basic energy substance (ATP) and genetic code.

SIGNS OF DEFICIENCY

Weakness, anorexia, bone pain. Prolonged use of antacids may cause deficiency.

SOURCES

Meat, fish, poultry, whole grains, nuts, cheese, phosphates in processed foods.

POTASSIUM

ESI: 1,875-5000 mg.

ROLE

Regulates heart beat, maintains body's fluid balance, stimulates nerve impulses, aid in muscle contraction.

SIGNS OF DEFICIENCY

Fatigue, muscle weakness, heart dysrhythmias.

SOURCES

Meat, bran, green leafy vegetables, potatoes, bananas, peanut butter, citrus fruits.

SELENIUM

ESI: 0.05-2 mg.

ROLE

Works with vitamin E to fight damage to cells caused by oxidation, maintains body growth.

SIGNS OF DEFICIENCY

Rare, deficiency may increase risk of cancer; however, research is inconclusive.

SOURCES

Seafood, meat, broccoli, onions, garlic, tomatoes, tuna, milk, egg yolk, whole grains.

SODIUM

ESI: 1,000-3,300 mg.

ROLE

Maintains fluid balance and the passage of substances in and out of cells, aids in functioning of nerves and muscles.

SIGNS OF DEFICIENCY

Deficiency is rare.   Muscle cramps, weakness, nausea, diarrhea.

SOURCES

Table salt, soy sauce, seafood, cured meats, cheese, processed foods.

ZINC

RDA: 15 mg.

ROLE

Maintains growth of sexual organs, production of essential enzymes, prostate function in men.

SIGNS OF DEFICIENCY

Deterioration of immune response, decreased wound healing.

SOURCES

Shellfish, meat, liver, eggs.

FOOD EXCHANGE LISTS

The food exchange list can be used for planning meals for the diabetic patient. In the exchange list foods are divided into six groups according to the amount of carbohydrates, proteins, fats and calories the food contains.

The foods within each of the six lists contains about the same amount of carbohydrates, proteins, and fats. In other words, all choices within a list are about equal. Any food on the list can be exchanged for any other food on the same list.

This chart shows the nutrients per serving from each exchange.

Exchange List	Carbohydrates (grams)	Protein (grams)	Fat (grams)	Calories
Starch/bread	15	3	trace	80
Meat				
Lean	0	7	3	55
Medium fat	0	7	5	75
High fat	0	7	8	100
Vegetable	5	2	0	25
Fruit	15	0	0	60
Milk				
Skim	12	8	trace	90
Low-fat	12	8	5	120
Whole	12	8	8	150
Fat	0	0	5	45

STARCH/BREAD LIST

As a general rule one serving equals:
1/2 cup cereal, grain or pasta
1 ounce of bread
1/2 cup starchy vegetables

BREADS

Bagel	1/2
Bread sticks	2
Croutons, low fat	1 cup
English muffin	1/2
Frankfurter or hamburger bun	1/2
Pita, 6 in. diameter	1/2
Plain roll, small	1
Raisin, unfrosted	1 slice
Rye, pumpernickel	1 slice
Tortilla, 6 in. diameter	1
White (incuding French, Italian)	1 slice
Whole wheat	1 slice
Dried bread crumbs	3 Tbsp

CEREALS/GRAINS/PASTA

Bran cereals, concentrated	1/3 cup

(such as Bran Buds, All Bran)

Bran cereals, flaked	1/2 cup
Bulgur (cooked)	1/2 cup
Cooked cereals	1/2 cup
Cornmeal	3 1/2 Tbsp
Grapenuts	3 Tbsp
Grits (cooked)	1/2 cup
Other ready-to-eat unsweetened cereals	3/4 cup
Pasta (cooked)	1/2 cup
Puffed cereal	1 1/2 cup
Rice, white or brown (cooked)	1/3 cup
Shredded wheat	1/2 cup
Wheat germ	3 Tbsp

DRIED BEANS/PEAS/LENTILS

Beans and peas (cooked, such as kidney, white, split, blackeyed)	1/3 cup
Lentils (cooked)	1/3 cup
Baked beans	1/4 cup

STARCHY VEGETABLES

Corn	1/2 cup
Corn on cob, 6 in. long	1
Lima beans	1/2 cup
Peas, green (canned or frozen)	1/2 cup
Potato, baked	1 small
Potato, mashed	1/2 cup
Squash, winter (acorn, butternut)	3/4 cup
Yam, sweet potato, plain	1/3 cup
Pumpkin	3/4 cup
Parsnips	2/3 cup

CRACKERS/SNACKS

Animal crackers	8
Graham crackers	3
Melba toast	5 slices
Oyster crackers	24

Popcorn (popped, no fat added)	3 cups
Pretzels	3/4 cup
Rye crisp	4
Saltine crackers	6
Whole wheat crackers	2-4 slices

PREPARED FOODS FOR BREAD EXCHANGES

(Count as 1 starch/bread serving, plus 1 fat serving)

Biscuit, 2 1/2 in. diameter	1
Chow mein noodles	1/2 cup
Corn bread, 2 in. cube	1
Cracker, round butter type	6
French fried potatoes	10
Muffin, plain, small	1
Pancake, 4 in. diameter	2
Stuffing, bread	1/4 cup
Taco shell, 6 in. diameter	2
Waffle, 4 1/2 in. square	1
Whole wheat crackers	4-6
Potato or corn chips	15
(count as 2 fat exchanges)	

MEAT LIST

Generally, one ounce of meat equals to one meat exchange. Meat should be weighed after removing bones and after cooking.

- Four ounces of raw meat equals to three ounces cooked. Some examples of meat portions are:

- chicken leg or thigh equals 2 ounces, or 2 exchanges,

- 1/2 cup cottage cheese or tuna equals 2 ounces, or 2 exchanges,

- 1 small hamburger equals 3 ounces, or 3 exchanges,

- 1/2 whole chicken breast equals 3 ounces, or 3 exchanges,

- 1 unbreaded fish filet equals 3 ounces, or 3 exchanges.

Because meat varies widely in fat content the meat list is divided into three categories: lean meat, medium-fat meat, and high-fat meat.

LEAN MEAT AND SUBSTITUTES

(Each serving is equal to one exchange)
Beef:

Round, sirloin, tenderloin	1 oz
Pork:	
Lean pork, tenderloin, ham, Canadian bacon	1 oz
Veal:	
All cuts, except veal cutlet	1 oz
Poultry:	
Chicken, turkey, Cornish hen (without skin)	1 oz
Fish:	
All fresh and frozen fish	1 oz
Crab, lobster, scallops, shrimp,	2 oz
Clams (fresh or canned in water)	2 oz
Oysters	6 medium
Tuna (canned in water)	1/4 cup
Herring (uncreamed or smoked)	1 oz

WILD GAME:

Venison, rabbit, squirrel,	1 oz
Pheasant, duck, goose (without skin)	1 oz

CHEESE:

Cottage cheese	1/4 cup
Grated parmesan	2 Tbsp
Diet cheeses (with less than 55 calories per ounce)	1 oz

OTHER:

95% fat-free luncheon meat	1 oz
Egg whites	3 whites
Egg substitutes with less than 55 calories per 1/4 cup	1/4 cup

MEDIUM-FAT AND SUBSTITUTES
BEEF:

Most beef products fall into this category. 1 oz
Examples: all ground beef, roast (rib,
  chuck, rump), steak (cubes, Porterhouse,
  T-bone), and meatloaf.

PORK:

Most pork products fall into this category. 1 oz
Examples: chops, loin roast, Boston butt,
  cutlets.

LAMB:

Most lamb products fall into this category 1 oz
Examples: chops, leg, and roast.

POULTRY:

Chicken (with skin), domestic duck or   1 oz
  goose (well-drained of fat), ground
  turkey.

FISH:

Tuna (canned in oil and drained)   1/4 cup
Salmon (canned)   1/4 cup

CHEESE:

Skim or part-skim milk cheeses, such as:
  Ricotta   1/4 cup
  Mozzarella   1 oz
  Diet cheeses (with 56-80 calories per oz) 1 oz

OTHER:

86% fat-free luncheon meat   1 oz
Egg (high in cholesterol, limit to 3 per   1
  week)
Egg substitutes   1/4 cup
Tofu   4 oz
Liver, heart, kidney, sweetbreads   1 oz
  (high in cholesterol)

HIGH-FAT MEAT AND SUBSTITUTES

Remember, these items are high in saturated fat, cholesterol, and calories, and should be used only three times per week. (One exchange is equal to any one of the following items)

BEEF:

Most USDA Prime cuts of beef, such as ribs corned beef.	1 oz

PORK:

Spareribs, ground pork, pork sausage (patty or link)	1 oz

LAMB:

Patties (ground lamb)	1 oz

FISH:

Any fried fish product	1 oz

CHEESE:

All regular cheeses, such as American, Blue, Cheddar, Monterey, Swiss	1 oz

OTHER:

Luncheon meat, such as bologna, salami, pimento loaf	1 oz
Sausage, such as Polish, Italian	1 oz
Knockwurst, smoked	1 oz
Bratwurst	1 oz
Frankfurter (turkey or chicken)	1 frank
Peanut butter (contains unsaturated fat)	1 Tbsp
Count as one high-fat meat plus one fat exchange: Frankfurter (beef, pork, or combination)	1 frank

FRESH, FROZEN, AND UNSWEETENED CANNED FRUIT

Apple	1
Applesauce (unsweetened)	1/2 cup
Apricots	4
Apricots (canned)	1/2 cup or 4 halves
Banana	1/2
Blackberries (raw)	3/4 cup
Blueberries (raw)	3/4 cup
Cantaloupe	1/3 melon or 1 cup cubes
Cherries	12
Cherries (canned)	1/2 cup
Figs	2
Fruit cocktail (canned)	1/2 cup
Grapefruit (medium)	1/2
Grapefruit (segments)	3/4 cup
Grapes	15
Honeydew melon	1/8 melon
Nectarines	1
Orange	1
Peach	1
Peaches (canned)	1/2 cup
Pear	1 small
Pears (canned)	1/2 cup
Pineapple (fresh)	3/4 cup
Pineapple (canned)	1/3 cup
Plum	2
Raspberries	1 cup
Strawberries	1 1/4 cup
Watermelon (cubes)	1 1/4 cup

DRIED FRUIT

Apples	4 rings
Apricots	7 halves

Dates	3 small
Figs	2 small
Prunes	4 small
Raisins	2 Tbsp

FRUIT JUICE

Apple juice/cider	1/2 cup
Cranberry juice/cocktail	1/3 cup
Grapefruit juice	1/2 cup
Grape juice	1/3 cup
Orange juice	1/2 cup
Pineapple juice	1/2 cup
Prune juice	1/3 cup

SKIM AND VERY LOWFAT MILK

Skim milk	1 cup
1% milk	1 cup
1/2% milk	1 cup
Low-fat buttermilk	1 cup
Evaporated skim milk	1/2 cup
Dry nonfat milk	1/3 cup
Plain, nonfat yogurt	8 oz

LOWFAT MILK

| 2% milk | 1 cup |
| Plain, lowfat yogurt | 8 oz |

WHOLE MILK

Whole milk	1 cup
Evaporated whole milk	1/2 cup
Whole plain yogurt	8 oz

UNSATURATED FATS

Avocado	1/8 medium
Margarine	1 tsp
Margarine, diet	1 Tbsp
Mayonnaise	1 tsp
Mayonnaise, reduced-calorie	1 Tbsp

NUTS AND SEEDS

Almonds, dry roasted	6 whole
Cashews, dry roasted	1 Tbsp
Pecans	2 whole
Peanuts	20 small or 10 large
Walnuts	2 whole
Other nuts	1 Tbsp
Seeds, pine nuts, sunflower (without shells)	1 Tbsp
Pumpkin seeds	2 tsp
Oils (corn, cottonseed, safflower, soybean, sunflower, olive, peanut)	1 tsp
Olives	10 small or 5 large
Salad dressing, mayonnaise-type	2 tsp
Salad dressing, mayonnaise-type reduced-calorie	1 Tbsp
Salad dressing	1 Tbsp
Salad dressing, reduced-calorie (2 Tbsp of low-calorie salad dressing is a free food)	2 Tbsp

SATURATED FATS

Butter	1 tsp
Bacon	1 slice
Coconut, shredded	2 Tbsp
Coffee whitener, liquid	2 Tbsp
Coffee whitener, powder	4 tsp
Cream (light, half and half)	2 Tbsp
Cream, sour	2 Tbsp
Cream (heavy, whipping)	1 Tbsp
Cream cheese	1 Tbsp
Salt pork	1/4 oz

FREE FOODS
DRINKS:

Bouillon or broth, without fat
Carbonated drinks, sugar free
Carbonated water
Club soda
Cocoa powder, unsweetened
(1 Tbsp)
Coffee/tea
Drink mixes, sugar-free

NONSTICK PAN SPRAY
FRUIT:

Cranberries, unsweetened   1/2 cup
Rhubarb, unsweetened   1/2 cup

VEGETABLES:

(raw, 1 cup)
Cabbage
Celery
Cucumber
Green onion
Hot peppers
Mushrooms
Radishes
Zucchini

SALAD GREENS:

Endive
Escarole
Lettuce
Romaine
Spinach

SWEET SUBSTITUTES:

Candy, hard, sugar-free
Gelatin, sugar-free

Gum, sugar-free
Jam/jelly, sugar-free
Pancake syrup, sugar-free
Sugar substitutes
Whipped topping

CONDIMENTS:

Catsup
Horseradish
Mustard
Pickles, dill, unsweetened
Salad dressing, low-calorie
Taco sauce
Vinegar

SEASONING:

Basil (fresh)
Celery seeds
Cinnamon
Chili powder
Chives
Curry
Dill
Flavoring extracts
(vanilla, almond, walnut,
peppermint, butter, lemon)
Garlic
Garlic powder
Herbs
Hot pepper sauce
Kitchen bouquet
Lemon
Lemon juice
Lemon pepper
Lime
Lime juice
Maple extract

Mint
Monosodium glutamate (MSG)
Onion powder
Oregano
Paprika
Parsley
Pepper
Pimento
Salt
Salt substitutes
Sesame seeds
Spices
Soy sauce
Soy sauce, low sodium
Tabasco sauce
Thyme
Vanilla extract
Vinegar
Wine, used in cooking (1/4 cup)
Worcestershire sauce

HOSPITAL DIETS

Diet	Foods Allowed	Precautions and Restrictions
Clear Liquid	Broth, bouillon, gelatin, tea, 7-Up	Serve at room temperature
Full Liquid	Any food on clear liquid diet and plain ice cream, sherbert, pudding, custard, yogurt, milk, milkshakes, eggnog, refined cooked cereals	Any food that will liquify at room temperature
Mechanical Soft	Regular diet that is chopped or pureed as required by the individual	Must be easy to swallow and digest
Regular or House	An ordinary diet, usually patient chooses own menu	No restrictions except personal preferences
Bland	Milk is a principle ingredient	Fatty foods, chocolate, citrus juices, highly seasoned foods, caffeine, alcohol
High Fiber	Fruits, vegetables, grains	No restrictions
Low Fiber	Milk, fruit juices, meats	Whole grains, cereals, fruits, vegetables
Low Protein	30-60 grams per day	Meat, fish, poultry, eggs, milk, cheese, beans
High Protein	More than 80 grams per day. Meat, eggs, cheese, beans, fish, poultry	No restrictions

Diet	Foods Allowed	Precautions and Restrictions
Low Purine	Regular diet with restrictions	Sardines, shrimp, liver, meat extracts, beans, peas
Gluten-free	Regular diet with restrictions	Wheat, oats, rye, barley
High Carbohydrate	Fruits, vegetables, grains, cereals, rice, pasta	No restrictions
Low Fat, Low Cholesterol	Fruits, vegetables, whole grains, cereals, beans, rice, fish, poultry, turkey	Marbled meats, any meat with skin, fried foods, pastry, cakes, chocolate, egg yolks, cheese
Low Sodium	2-4 grams per day. Regular diet with restrictions	Salt, catsup, soy sauce, cured meats, canned foods, cheese, peanut butter, biscuit mixes, pickles, olives, instant cooked cereals
Low Potassium	Reduction of average 6 gram to 2 gram. Regular diet with restrictions	Milk, meat, poultry, apricots, banana, cantaloupe, oranges, prunes, raisins, beans, potatoes, spinach, sweet potato, tomatoes
High Calcium	More than 1000 mg. per day. Milk, cheese, vitamin supplement	Must have adequate amount of vitamin D for absorption

Diet	Foods Allowed	Precautions and Restrictions
Diabetic Diets	Recommended distribution of calories: 60 percent carbohydrate, 20-30 percent protein, 20-30 percent fat	Simple carbohydrates such as candy, cake, pastries, fruits usually limited to 4 per day.

DIETARY GUIDELINES

The Surgeon General recommends the following dietary guidelines for the promotion of health and prevention of disease.

1. Eat a variety of foods.
   A well-balanced diet including the Basic Four will supply the nutrients needed for health. No one food or one diet can provide all nutritional requirements.

2. Maintain ideal body weight.
   Avoid high-calorie, low-nutrient foods such as sweets, fats, and alcohol. Increase and/or include physical exercise.

3. Avoid saturated fat and cholestorol.
   Eat lean meat, poultry, and fish while limiting egg yolks and organ meats. Avoid rich desserts with heavy cream and chocolate. Broil and bake to avoid frying meats. Fat intake should be 30% or less of the total intake of calories. Cholesterol intake should be less than 3000 milligrams daily.

4. Eat foods high in fiber, starch, and complex carbohydrates.
   Whole grains, nuts, beans, fruits and vegetables should make up the bulk of the diet.

5. Avoid sugar and salt.

    Limit intake at simple sugars such as honey, sugar, candy, soft drinks. Limit intake of foods high in salt such as processed foods, smoked and cured meats, and snack foods.

    Salt intake should be six grams, or less, per day.

6. Drink alcohol only in moderation.

    A limit of two alcoholic drinks is recommended. A 12 oz. beer, 4 oz. of wine, or 1 oz. of hard liquor is equal to one drink. Pregnant women should not drink alcohol.

7. Maintain adequate intake of iron, calcium, and flouride. Eat foods high in these minerals. While supplements are recommended, do not exceed RDA allowances.

Source: Adapted from the Surgeon General's Report on Nutrition and Health: Summary and Recommendations, DHS publication No. 88- 50211 (Washington, D.C.: Government Printing Office, 1989).

Metropolitan Life Insurance Company

Height & Weight Chart

In 1983 the Metropolitan Life Insurance Company devised a height-weight scale that has become a standard.

WOMEN

Height Ft. In.	Small	Frame Medium	Large
4 10	102-111	109-121	118-131
4 11	103-113	111-123	120-134
5 0	104-115	113-126	122-137
5 1	106-118	115-129	125-140
5 2	108-121	118-132	128-143

Height Ft. In.	Small	Frame Medium	Large
5 3	111-124	121-135	131-147
5 4	114-127	124-138	134-151
5 5	117-130	127-141	137-155
5 6	120-133	130-144	140-159
5 7	123-136	133-147	143-163
5 8	126-139	136-150	146-167
5 9	129-142	139-153	149-170
5 10	132-145	142-156	152-173
5 11	135-148	145-159	155-176
6 0	138-151	148-162	158-179

MEN

Height Ft. In.	Small	Frame Medium	Large
5 2	128-134	131-141	138-150
5 3	130-136	133-143	140-153
5 4	132-138	135-145	142-156
5 5	134-140	137-148	144-160
5 6	136-142	139-151	146-164
5 7	138-145	142-154	149-168
5 8	140-148	145-157	152-172
5 9	142-151	148-160	155-176
5 10	144-154	151-163	158-180
5 11	146-157	154-166	161-184
6 0	149-160	157-170	164-188
6 1	152-164	160-174	168-192
6 2	155-168	164-178	172-197
6 3	158-172	167-182	176-202
6 4	162-176	171-187	181-207

GLASGOW COMA SCALE

The Glasgow coma scale is an invaluable assessment to for monitoring neurologic dysfunction. When using the GCS, determine the score in each of the three tests and add all three scores. A total of 13-15 indicates moderates minor dysfunction, a score of 9-13 indicates moderate dysfunction, and a score of less than 8 indicates a neurologic crisis.

GLASGOW COMA SCALE

EYES OPEN

Spontaneously	4
To Speech	3
To Pain	2
No Response	1

VERBAL RESPONSE

Oriented/Talking	5
Disoriented/Talking	4
Words Inappropriate	3
Incomprehensible	2
No Response	1

MONITOR RESPONSE

Obeys Command	6
Localizes Pain	5
Flexion: Withdrawal	4
Decorticate: Flexion	3
Decerebrate: Rigidity	2
No Response	1

NEUROCHECKS

Neurological checks are frequently performed on many hospitalized patients. Neuro-checks are usually documented on a separate flow sheet, but the following check points are important to a thorough assessment.

Consciousness

Alert (awake, responds appropriately)

Lethargic (sleepy, but arouses easily)

Obtuned (responds appropriately, but difficult to arouse)

Stuporous (responds to painful stimuli, never completely alert)

Semicomatose (responds to painful stimuli, relfex movements only)

Comatose (no response, no reflex)

Orientation

Person

Place

Time

Situation

Judgment

Coherent

Thoughts distorted

Verbal response appropriate

Memory

Recent

Past

Remote

Affect

Blunted
Alert
Pleasant
Restricted

Speech

Aphasia
Dysphasia
Articulate
Appropriate

Pain

Reaction to stimul
Reaction to painful stimuli

Pupil Assessment

+Reactive
-Nonreactive
-Sluggish

Neurovascular

Compromised points
External Restrictions (such as cast, traction, restraints)
Adequate ROM

Motor

Decerebrate
Decordicate

MENTAL STATUS ASSESSMENT

A mental status assessment is necessary for any patient in the hospital, especially if their health status is psychologically sensitive. Patients who are diagnosed with cancer, cerebrovascular accident or severe injuries are just a few examples of patients who need the special attention that a mental status assessment offers.

Name
Age
Sex
General Appearance
    Appropriate/neat
    Inappropriate/unkept
    Overly meticulous
    Bizarre
    Posture/gait
    Bodily mannerisms
Behavior/Attitude
    Affect/emotional state
    Cooperative
    Pleasant
    Withdrawn
    Indifferent
    Hostile
    Euphoric
    Suspicious
    Naive
Content of Thought
    Spontaneous replies
    Preoccupied

Ideas of reference
Looseness of association
Delusions
Hallucinations (auditory, visual)
Illusions
Grandiosity
Somatic complaints
Suicidal thoughts
Suicidal plans
Obsessions
Compulsions
Phobias
Cognitive Functioning
Insight
Awareness of self
Awareness of others
Awareness of situation
Orientation
Memory: recent, remote
Abstract thought process
Concrete thought process
General intelligence level
Judgment
Decision-making skills
Problem-solving skills
Intellectual functioning/knowledge base
Ability to Cope with Anxiety
Defense mechanisms
Accepts responsibility for actions
Stress-crisis cycle

General Response Pattern during Interview
    Appropriate
    Cooperative
    Trusting
    Anxious
    Angry
    Indifferent
    Withdrawn

Folstein's Mini-Mental Status Exam

A mental status exam should be done on every patient.
This mini-mental status exam developed by Folstein is a
simple, practical, widely-used test that can be administered
in just a few minutes. It is a useful test that can be done
frequently, even daily, to track a patient's deterioration or
recovery. It is most often utilized with the geriatric,
stroke, and AIDS patient. The higher the score, the
higher the patient's level of functioning.

Patient_____

Examiner_____ Date_____

Maximum

Score	Score	ORIENTATION
5	_____	What is the date? (year, season, day, month)
5	_____	Where are we? (state, town, hospital, floor)
		REGISTRATION
3	_____	Name 3 objects: 1 second to say each. Then ask the patient all 3 after you have said them. Give one point for each correct answer.

Then repeat them until he learns all
three. Count trials and record.
Trials _____

ATTENTION AND CALCULATION

5   _____   Serial 7's. One point for each
             correct. Stop after 5 answers.
             Alternatively, spell "world"
             backwards.

RECALL

3   _____   Ask for the 3 objects repeated
             above. Give 1 point for each
             correct answer.

LANGUAGE

9   _____   Name a pencil, and watch.
             Repeat the following: "No ifs,
             and's or but's." (1 point)
             Follow a 3-stage command:
             "Take a paper in your right hand,
             fold it in half, and put it on
             the floor." (3 points)

             Read and obey the following:

1   _____   CLOSE YOUR EYES (1 point)
1   _____   WRITE A SENTENCE (1 point)
1   _____   COPY DESIGN   (1 point)

    _____   TOTAL SCORE

ASSESS level of consciousness along a continuum:

| Alert | Drowsy | Stupor | Coma |

PSYCHIATRIC ASSESSMENT

A psychiatric assessment differs from a mental health status assessment in that a psychiatric assessment is performed only on patients who have a psychiatric diagnosis. Many patients have a secondary psychiatric diagnosis, such as depression.

Psychiatric Assessment Form

Response to Anxiety

Defense mechanisms are utilized to decrease anxiety, and coping strategies are tasks oriented to reality. For example, denial is a coping strategy. The way in which these strategies are used determines whether behavior is healthy or unhealthy.

What to Assess:

Level of Anxiety
  Mild
  Moderate
  Severe
  Panic
 Physical Signs and Symptoms
  Palpitations
  Diaphoresis
  Increased pulse
  Increased respirations
  Increased blood pressure
  Tendency to worry
  Inability to concentrate
  Effective use of defense mechanisms

Assessment Questions:

What stressful events have you experienced in
   the past?

How have you coped in the past?

How do you cope with stress on the job?

How do you cope with stress at home?

Interpersonal skills

Interpersonal relationships cause anxiety, threaten self-
esteem and hold the risk of rejection. The pattern of
recurrent interpersonal relationships has a dramatic impact
on an individual's mental health.

What to Assess:

Anger

Hostility

Bitterness

Contempt

Suspiciousness

Controlling

Cooperative

Trusting

Withdrawal

Isolation

Avoidance

Submissiveness

Spontaneous

Dependent

Difficulty in communications

Assessment Questions:

With whom do you share your good feelings?

With whom do you share your bad feelings?

Do you have a significant other with whom you feel free to talk?

How do you get along with co-workers?

How do you get along with your family?

Do you feel comfortable in most social situations?

Do you avoid many social events?

Are you appropriately assertive with others?

Who is your strongest support system?

Spirit of Optimism

People strive first to meet their basic needs then seek to grow, change and reach their optimal potential. The motivating key to reach this potential is some degree of optimism or hope that their goals are obtainable.

What to Assess:

Hopelessness

Helplessness

Inappropriate laughter

Crying

Blunted affect

Despondency

Detachment

Assessment Questions:

How could things be better for you?

What can you do to bring about these positive changes?

Are you willing to take risks for change that would make you happy?

Do you have joy in your life?

What is the source?

What motivates you?

Tell me how you spend your time during a
typical day.

Language/Nonverbal Behavior

Behavior is expressed both verbally and nonverbally.
What the patient says reflects what he is feeling, thinking,
and how he is reacting to certain situations. Nonvebal
behavior is also quite reflective, and it is important that
verbal and nonverbal are congruent.

What to Assess:

Slurred speech

Inappropriate speech

Unusual mannerisms

Rigidity

Fidgeting

Poor hygiene

Unkept appearance

Arrogant

Histrionic

Incongruence between speech and behavior

Assessment Questions:

Note any unusual gestures by the patient.

Is rigid behavior exhibited?

Describe the patient's affect.

How is the verbal and nonverbal behavior
incongruent?

Self-awareness

Identification of feelings is a critical component in
self-awareness and is significantly enhanced when the

patient associates that feelings and actions are intimately interwined with one's behavior. Insight is difficult to develop and often requires therapy.

What to Assess:

Insight
Self-awareness
Judgment
Guilt
Remorse
Fear of failure
Fear of success
Paranoia
Passive-aggressive personality
Grief reaction
Stress-crisis cycle*

*The stress-crisis cycle is set up when a person cannot function or accomplish goals unless they are under intense stress. This is usually caused by procrastination or self-imposed goals which may be unrealistic.

Assessment Questions:

What are you feeling now?
How do you react when you are angry?
How do you react when you depressed?
Do you procrastinate to the point of crisis?
Do you function daily in a stress-crisis cycle?

Thought Processes

Thought processes are monitored by the expression of reason and logic. When a patient expresses irrational thoughts, there is a disturbance at both conscious and unconscious levels.

What to Assess:

Orientation
Person
Place
Time
Situation
Irrelevant responses
Incoherent responses
Conceptual disorganization
Grandiosity
Hallucinations (perception of things not present)
Delusions (a false belief)
Illusions (misperceptions of real stimulus)

Assessment Questions:

What is your name?
What day is it?
Where are you now?
What's going on here and now?
Are your thoughts disturbing you?
Do you hear voices?
Do you see things that are not there?

Strengths and power

Focusing on personal assets and strengths gives a balanced, holistic view of the patient's insight and ability to cope.

What to Assess:

Strengths
Job skills
Talents/hobbies

Past adjustment to stress
Support systems
Ability to communicate
Appearance

Assessment Questions:

What do you do well?
What do you enjoying doing?
How have you successfully coped in the past?
What do you like best about yourself?
What do you like least about yourself?

Physical Symptoms

There are many links between physical and mental health. A physical symptom is often symbolic of unresolved psychological stressors or feelings. Physical illnesses such as ulcers, heart attacks and headaches are more often accepted as an illness than repressed anger, rage and guilt.

What to Assess:

Headaches
Gastrointestinal disorders
Chest pain
High blood pressure
Weight
Appetite
Sexual activity
Body image
General health
Sleep disturbance
Energy level

Assessment Questions:

Describe your general physical health.

What body reactions do you notice when you are stressed, angry or depressed?

Can you associate certain physical symptoms to certain stressors?

Do you tend to ignore your body during psychological crises?

Incompetence of Personality

Instability in interpersonal relationships, impulsiveness and unpredictable behavior may indicate an inadequate personality. This patient lacks a sense of responsibility to others and has difficulty finding their role in society. They are bored, angry and discontent. They have no concept of setting and accomplishing goals, and they have no value system on which to base their actions.

What to Assess:

Irritability
Anger
Forgetfulness
Mood swings
Boredom
Compulsiveness
Unsatisfying relationships
Inability to adjust to situations

Assessment Questions:

Do you complete routine tasks without assistance?

Do you display interest in surroundings and in others?

Do you laugh or joke appropriately?

Do you initiate communication?

Do you often exhibit lack of control, particularly
outbursts of anger?

The Addictive Personality

The addictive personality uses chemicals to escape from
reality into what becomes for them a pleasureable existence.
They are constantly seeking a recreation of the first
rewarding feelings they experienced when they used drugs
and alcohol. They seek to fulfill a fantasy when they cannot
accept the reality of their life.

What to Assess:

Nervousness

Irritability

Aggressiveness

Low frustration levels

Anger

Mood swings

Depressive episodes

Indifference

Helplessness

Antagonistic attitude

Bizarre behaviors

Unpredictable behavior

Euphoria

Grandiosity

Distortion of reality

Suicidal ideations

Assessment Questions

Do you resent others?

Are you secretive about your activities?

Do you make excessive excuses for your actions?

Do you experience mood swings?

BECK DEPRESSION INVENTORY

NAME _____ DATE _____

On this questionnaire are groups of statements. Please read each group of statements carefully. Then pick out the one statement in each group which best describes the way you have been feeling the past week, including today. Circle the number beside the statement you picked. If several statements in the group seem to apply equally well, circle each one. Be sure to read all the statements in each group before making your choice.

1   0   I do not feel sad.
    1   I feel sad.
    2   I am sad all the time and I can't snap out of it.
    3   I am so sad of being unhappy that I can't stand it.

2   0   I am not particularly discouraged about the future.
    1   I feel discouraged about the future.
    2   I feel I have nothing to look forward to.
    3   I feel that the future is hopeless and that things cannot improve.

3 0 I do not feel like a failure.
   1 I feel I have failed more than the average person.
   2 As I look back on my life, all I can see is a lot of failures.
   3 I feel I am a complete failure as a person.

4 0 I get as much satisfaction out of things as I used to.
   1 I don't enjoy things the way I used to.
   2 I don't get real satisfaction out of anything anymore.
   3 I am dissatisfied or bored with everything.

5 0 I don't feel particularly guilty.
   1 I feel guilty a good part of the time.
   2 I feel quite guilt most of the time.
   3 I feel guilty all of the time.

6 0 I don't feel I am being punished.
   1 I feel I may be punished.
   2 I expect to be punished.
   3 I feel I am being punished.

7 0 I don't feel disappointed in myself.
   1 I am disappointed in myself.
   2 I am disgusted with myself.
   3 I hate myself.

8 0 I don't feel I am any worse than anybody else.
   1 I am critical of myself for my weaknesses or mistakes.
   2 I blame myself all the time for my faults.
   3 I blame myself for everything bad that happens.

9 0 I don't have any thoughts of killing myself.
 1 I have thoughts of killing myself, but I would not carry them out.
 2 I would like to kill myself.
 3 I would kill myself if I had the chance.

10 0 I don't cry any more than usual.
 1 I cry more now than I used to.
 2 I cry all the time now.
 3 I used to be able to cry, but now I can't cry even though I want to.

11 0 I am no more irritated now than I ever am.
 1 I get annoyed or irritated more easily than I used to.
 2 I feel irritated all the time now.
 3 I don't get irritated at all by the things that used to irritate me.

12 0 I have not lost interest in other people.
 1 I am less interested in other people than I used to be.
 2 I have lost most of my interest in other people.
 3 I have lost all of my interest in other people.

13 0 I make decisions about as well as I ever could.
 1 I put off making decisions more than I used to.
 2 I have greater difficulty in making decisions than before.
 3 I can't make decisions at all anymore.

14 0 I don't feel I look any worse than I used to.
 1 I am worried that I am looking old or unattractive.
 2 I feel that there are permanent changes in my appearance that make me look unattractive.
 3 I believe that I look ugly.

15 0 I can work about as well as before.

   1 It takes an extra effort to get started at doing something.

   2 I have to push myself very hard to do anything.

   3 I can't do any work at all.

16 0 I can sleep as well as usual.

   1 I don't sleep as well as I used to.

   2 I wake up 1-2 hours earlier than usual and find it hard to get back to sleep.

   3 I wake up several hours earlier than I used to and cannot get back to sleep.

17 0 I don't get more tired than usual.

   1 I get tired more easily than I used to.

   2 I get tired from doing almost anything.

   3 I am too tired to do anything.

18 0 My appetite is no worse than usual.

   1 My appetite is not as good as it used to be.

   2 My appetite is much worse now.

   3 I have no appetite at all anymore.

19 0 I haven't lost much weight, if any, lately.

   1 I have lost more than 5 pounds.

   2 I have lost more than 10 pounds.

   3 I have lost more than 15 pounds.

     I am purposely trying to lose weight by eating less.

     Yes _____   No _____

20 0   I am no more worried about my health than usual.

    1   I am worried about physical problems such as aches and pains; or upset stomach; or constipation.

    2   I am very worried about physical problems and it's hard to think of much else.

    3   I am so worried about my physical problems, that I cannot think about anything else.

21 0   I have not noticed any recent changed in my interest in sex.

    1   I am less interested in sex than I used to be.

    2   I am much less interested in sex now.

    3   I have lost interest in sex completely.

The Beck Depression Inventory is a self-administered test that is easily scored. It assesses symptoms of depression that include poor concentration, suicidal thoughts, feelings of guilt, hopelessness, helplessness, loss of appetite and various physical symptoms. In scoring the 21 items, the maximum score is 63. A score of 11-16 indicates mild depression, 17-25 moderate depression and a score over 25 could be indicative of severe depression. This inventory should be utilized only as a guide in how a person is feeling and thinking. The results should be analyzed only by a professional.

Printed with permission from the Center for Cognitive Therapy.

DEFENSE MECHANISMS

Defense mechanisms, or coping strategies, are used to cope with anxiety. The use of some of these mechanisms are healthy, and some are unhealthy. Often these patterns of behavior operate at an unconscious level to block conscious awareness of threatening feelings.

COMPENSATION A person overemphasizes one aspect of the personality in an effort to make up for what they consider a deficiency in another aspect.

Example: An obese woman is obsessed about how her makeup and hair look. Or, a homely schoolgirl attempts to impress her peers by making straight A's.

CONVERSION The process of turning psychological conflicts into physical symptoms. The patient often realizes some secondary gain from the pain.

Example: A wife is told her husband is having an affair, and she starts having headaches. He calls through the day checking to see how she is feeling.

DENIAL Refusal to recognize or deal with reality. A protective mechanism utilized in traumatic situations when the person cannot comprehend the overwhelming onslaught of a tragedy.

Example: A mother refuses to participate in funeral arrangements after her child is killed in a car wreck.

Example: A man comes to the emergency room with chest pain, insisting he be treated only for indigestion, refusing to realize he may be having a heart attack.

DISPLACEMENT An unacceptable feeling, emotion, or reaction such as anger, is unconsciously discharged or transferred toward someone or something other than the source of the feeling.

Example: The man comes home angry because his boss chewed him out, and he kicks the dog.

IDENTIFICATION   The extreme imitation of another person who is feared or respected. Characteristics of the person being imitated is incorporated into the personality.

Example: A boy who idolizes his father tells his new friends his nickname is "Smokey." This is his father's nickname, not his.

INTELLECTUALIZATION   The use of rational explanations to justify unacceptable behavior or feelings.

Example: An executive who has just been admitted to a chemical dependency unit attempts to convince the other patients that he is different because of his professional and financial status.

INTROJECTION   The incorporation of another person's values into one's own lifestyle and philosophy.

Example: A college student follows his parents' instruction to abstain from casual sex.

RATIONALIZATION   The process of justifying one's behavior by using an excuse that is directed toward another person or situation. The reasons used to explain unacceptable behavior are often exaggerated and untrue.

Example: A student fails an exam and blames it on poor lectures by the instructor.

REACTION FORMATION Behavior that is directly opposite of the way the person actually feels. This is typically passive-aggressive behavior.

Example: A secretary is very nice and polite to her boss, but actually hates him.

REGRESSION Falling back into an earlier mode of behavior and feelings that is more comfortable and less demanding.

Example: A 6-year-old boy assumes a fetal position and starts wetting the bed after he is told his parents are getting a divorce.

REPRESSION The unconscious process of blocking painful or threatening thoughts, feelings, and experiences from the conscious so that the painful issues are not confronted or resolved.

Example: A woman who was sexually abused as a child blocks the experience from her conscious and is confused about her inability to response sexually to her husband.

SUBLIMATION Directing sexual or aggressive impulses into a more socially-accepted activity.

Example: The football star would like to have sex with his girlfriend, but puts all of his energy into playing the sport.

SUPPRESSION The conscious process of ignoring painful thoughts or impulses.

Example: A man agrees to go to marriage counseling with his wife and "forgets" to show up for the appointment.

UNDOING Words or behavior that attempt to annul actions that have met with disapproval or caused feelings of guilt.

Example: A husband goes on a drinking binge, and the next day sends his wife flowers.

LEVELS OF ANXIETY

MILD
Increased awareness
Stimulated toward action
Positively motivated
Slight increase in vital signs

MODERATE
Tension heightens
Perceptions and concentration decreases
Alert, but focus narrows
Slight increase in vital signs
Physical symptoms develop: Headache, urinary frequency, nausea, palpitations, restlessness

SEVERE
Perceptions become distorted
Intense feelings of dread or threat
Communication becoming distorted
More dramatic increases in vital signs, diarrhea, diaphoresis, palpitations, chest pain, vomiting

PANIC
Feelings of terror
Reality distorted
Unable to communicate
Combination of physical symptoms listed above with increased vital signs early in the panic stage, but may drop if intervention is not successful
Could be harmful to self and/or others

SIGNS AND SYMPTOMS OF DRUG ABUSE

Drug	Signs & Symptoms	Assessment
Alcohol	Slurred speech Unsteady gait Slow reflexes Impaired coordination No inhibitions Abnormal relaxation	Smell of alcohol Glazed eyes Headaches Giddish behavior

Complication: Accidents that result from impaired judgment
Overdose when mixed with drugs
Liver damage
Eventually all body organs will be damaged
Addiction

Drug	Signs & Symptoms	Assessment
Depressants Barbiturates Sedatives Tranquilizers	Decreased respirations Slowed heart rate Drowsiness Uncoordination May appear to be intoxicated	Sleep more than 10 hours Slurred speech Presence of pills without prescription labels Confused behavior

Complication: Overdose, especially when combined with alcohol
Rigidity or stiffness
Withdrawal which requires medical attention
Addiction

Marijuana
Reddened eyes
Dry mouth
Drowsiness
Lack of coordination
Lack of concentration
Euphoria
Craving sweets
Impulsiveness
Illusions

Paraphernalia
Altered vision and
auditory perception
Overestimations of
time and space
Talkative
Disorientation

Complication: Panic attacks
Impotence
Impaired memory, especially short-term
Addiction

Cocaine
Increased heart rate,
blood pressure
Intense euphoria
Extreme restlessness
Euphoria is followed
by depression

Paraphernalia:
glass
vials
pipes
white crystalline
powder
syringes
needle marks

Complication: Heart attack
Seizures
Addiction
Severe depression
Paranoid ideations

Hallucinogens
Acid
LSD
PCP
Mescaline

Obsession with detail
Mood swings
Panic attacks
Nausea and vomiting
Synaesthesia (seeing
sounds and smelling
colors)
Altered perceptions
Increased anxiety

Flushing
Vomiting
Cramping
Increased pulse
Muscle twitching
Hallucinations

Complication: Unpredictable, often dangerous behavior
Violence with PCP
Emotionally unstable

Inhalants	Dizziness	Odor of substance
Gasoline	Lack of coordination	Drowsiness
Glue	Uncontrolled behavior	Intoxication
Hair spray	Nausea and vomiting	
White out		
(correction fluid)		

Complication: Unconsciousness
Suffocation
CNS damage
Sudden death

Narcotics	Drowsiness	Needle marks, especially on arms
	Euphoria	Syringes
	No sensitivity to pain	Constricted or dilated pupils
	Watery eyes	Cold, clammy skin
	Runny eyes	
	Nausea, vomiting	

Complication: Addiction
Weight loss
Hepatitis
AIDS
Overdose

Stimulants	Alertness	Increased blood pressure
Speed	Hypertalkative	Weight loss
Uppers	Insomnia	Loss of sleep
Caffeine	Disorientation	Loss of appetite
Nicotine	Hallucinations	
Amphetamines		

Complication: Exhaustion
Addiction
Paranoia
Depression

SEVEN CARDINAL SIGNS OF DRUG ABUSE

1. Change in performance at work or school
2. Alterations in personal appearance
3. Change in attitude or mood swings
4. Withdrawal from family relationships
5. Friends who use drugs
6. New and unusual patterns of behavior
7. Defensive attitude concerning behavior

THE KATZ INDEX OF ACTIVITIES OF DAILY LIVING

The Katz Index of Activities of Daily Living is commonly used, especially with geriatric patients to assess functionly ability.   The tool can also assess deterioriation or progress in the patient who has problems with ADL. The tool is not scored, but serves as an assessment guide.

AREAS AND LEVELS OF ASSESSMENT IN THE KATZ INDEX OF INDEPENDENCE IN ACTIVITIES OF DAILY LIVING

BATHING
  Receives no assistance
  Receives assistance in bathing only one part
  Receives assistance in bathing more than one part

DRESSING
  Gets clothes and dresses without assistance
  Needs assistance in tying shoes only
  Needs assistance greater than above or stays undressed

TOILETING
  Needs no assistance
  Needs assistance only in getting to toilet room or in
    cleaning self
  Does not go to toilet room

TRANSFERRING
  Needs no assistance from another person
  Needs assistance with transferring
  Does not get out of bed

CONTINENCE

Continent

Occasional accident

Needs supervision, uses catheter, or is incontinent

FEEDING

Needs no assistance

Needs assistance in cutting meat or buttering bread

Needs more assistance or is tube or intravenously feed

SOCIAL ADJUSTMENT RATING SCALE

The Holmes-Rahe scale has become the guide by which modern stressors are measured. The research Holmes and Rahe produced using this scale indicates the amount of stress a person is under is directly related to his vulnerability to illness.

RANK	LIFE EVENT	LIFE CHANGE UNITS
1	Death of spouse	100
2	Divorce	73
3	Marital separation	65
4	Jail term	63
5	Death of close family member	63
6	Personal injury or illness	53
7	Marriage	50
8	Fired from job	47
9	Marital reconciliation	45
10	Retirement	45
11	Change in health of a family member	44

RANK	LIFE EVENT	LIFE CHANGE UNITS
12	Pregnancy	40
13	Sexual difficulties	39
14	Gain of new family member	39
15	Business readjustment	39
16	Change in financial state	38
17	Death of close friend	37
18	Change to different line of work	36
19	Change in number of arguments with spouse	35
20	Mortgage over $10,000	31
21	Foreclosure of mortgage or loan	30
22	Change in responsibilities at work	29
23	Son or daughter leaving home	29
24	Trouble with in-laws	29
25	Outstanding personal achievement	28
26	Spouse begins or stops work	26
27	Begin or end school	26
28	Change in living conditions	25
29	Revision of personal habits	24
30	Trouble with boss	23
31	Change in work hours or conditions	20
32	Change in residence	20
33	Change in school	20
34	Change in recreation	19
35	Change in church activities	19
36	Change in social activities	18
37	Mortgage or loan less than $10,000	17
38	Change in sleeping habits	16

RANK	LIFE EVENT	LIFE CHANGE UNITS
39	Change in number of family get-togethers	15
40	Change in eating habits	15
41	Vacation	13
42	Christmas	12
43	Minor violations of the law	11

The scoring:

1-149	Represents no significant life changes
150-199	Indicates mild life changes with 33% chance of illness
200-299	Indicates moderate changes with 50% chance of illness
Over 300	Indicates major life changes with 80% chance of illness.

CLINICAL VALUES
AND STANDARDS

CLINICAL VALUES AND STANDARDS

Table of Contents

BURN FORMULAS

Fluid Replacement in First 24 Hours

Fluid replacement must be calculated from the time of the burn, not from the time of admission. During the first 24-hour period, one half of the solution is administered during the first eight hours and the other half is equally divided over the next sixteen hours.

FORMULA NAME	ELECTRO-LYTE	COLLOID	WATER
BROOKE	Lactated Ringer's 1.5 ml x kg body weight x % TBSA. ** Example: 1.5 x 70 x 60=6,300 ml	0.5 ml x kg body weight x/TBSA. Example: 0.5 x 70 x 60=2,100 ml	2,000 ml D5W
MODIFIED BROOKE	Lactated Ringer's 2 ml x kg x % TBSA; up to 4 ml/ kg / %. Example: 2 X 70 X 60=8,400 ml	0	0

PARKLAND or BAXTER	Lactated Ringer's 4 ml x kg x % TBSA. Example: 4x 70 x 60= 16,800 ml Administer 1/2 total over first 8 hours (from time of burn), 1/4 total over second 8 hours, 1/4 total over third 8 hours	0	0

(TBSA-- Total Burn Surface Area)

** Examples are based on a 154 lb. (70 kg) person who has been burned over 60% of the body.

THE RULE OF NINES

In calculating Total Burn Surface Area (TBSA), the Rule of Nines is used. Percentages are designated for each area burned, then added for the TBSA.

USING THE "RULE OF NINES"

A nurse can quickly estimate the extent of an adult's burn with the "Rule of Nines." This method divides an adult's body surface area into percentages that equal 100%. To use this method, match the patient's burns to the body chart shown here, then add the percentages. The total is used in the formula to determine initial fluid replacement needs. (See chart on next page.)

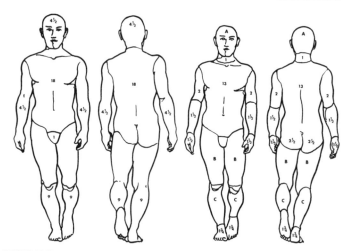

USING THE LUND AND BROWDER CHART

The "Rule of Nines" cannot be used for infants and children because the body section percentages differ from those of adults. For example, an infant's head accounts for 19% of total body surface area, compared to 9% for an adult. To determine the extent of an infant's or child's burns, use the Lund and Browder chart. This chart takes age differences into account.

Relative percentages of areas affected by growth

Front	At Birth	1 yr.	5 yrs.	10 yrs.
A: Half of head	9 1/2%	8 1/2%	6 1/2%	5 1/2%
B: Half of thigh	2 3/4%	3 1/4%	4%	4 1/4%
C: Half of leg	2 1/2%	2 1/2%	2 3/4%	3%
		15 yrs.		Adult
A: Half of head		4 1/2%		3 1/2%
B: Half of thigh		4 1/2%		4 3/4%
C: Half of leg		3 1/4%		3 1/2%

Estimating Burn Extent:

The Lund and Browder Chart (Children)

Determine the extent of an infant's burns by using this Lund and Browder chart, which estimates body surface area proportionate to the infant's or child's size and age.

Relative percentages of areas affected by growth

Back	At birth	Age 1	Age 5	Age 10
A: Half of head	9 1/2%	8 1/2%	6 1/2%	5 1/2%
B: Half of thigh	2 3/4%	3 1/4%	4%	4 1/4%
C: Half lower leg	2 1/2%	2 1/2%	2 3/4%	3%
		Age 15		
A: Half of head		4 1/2%		
B: Half of thigh		4 1/2%		
C: Half of lower leg		3 1/4%		

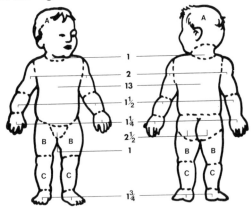

ABBREVIATIONS USED IN HEALTH CARE

These abbreviations are presented as a guide only, some hospitals do not accept all of these or use different ones than those presented here.

a	before
aa	of each
AB	abortion
abd	abdomen
ABGs	arterial blood gases
a.c.	before meals
ADA	American Diabetes Association
ADH	antidiuretic hormone
AKA	also known as
ad lib	as desired
AMA	against medical advice
amb	ambulation
ant	anterior
AP	anterior - posterior
AROM	active range of motion
ASA	acetylsalicylic acid, aspirin
ASAP	as soon as possible
ASHD	arteriosclerotic heart disease
BID	twice a day
BM	bowel movement
BMR	basal metabolic rate
BP	blood pressure
BPH	benign prostatic hypertrophy
BS	blood sugar
BUN	blood urea nitrogen

Bx	biopsy
c	with
cap	capsules
C	celsius (centigrade)
Ca	cancer
cath	catherization
CC	chief complaint
cc	cubic centimeter
CBC	complete blood count
CHF	congestive heart failure
cm	centimeter
CNS	central nervous system
CO2	carbon dioxide
c/o	complains of
COPD	chronic obstuctive pulmonary disease
CPAP	continuous positive airway pressure
CPR	cardiopulmonary resuscitation
C-section	cesarean section
CSF	cerebrospinal fluid
CVA	cerebrovascular accident
CVP	central venous pressure
D5W	5% glucose in water
D&C	dilatation & curettage
DC	discontinued
dl	deciliter
D.M.	diabetes mellitus
DOA	dead on arrival
DOB	date of birth
dr	dram
dsg	dressing
dx	diagnosis

ECG	electrocardiogram
EEG	electroencephalogram
elix	elixir
EENT	ear, eye, nose & throat
F	fahrenheit
FBS	fasting blood sugar
FIO2	inspired oxygen concentration
FHS	follicle - stimulating hormone
fx	fracture
gal	gallon
gm or G	gram
gr	grain
gtts	drops
GI	gastrointestinal
GU	genitourinary
Gyn	gynecology
H	hypodermically
H2O	water
Hct	hematocrit
Hgb	hemoglobin
HOB	head of bed
hr	hour
hs	at bedtime
Hx	history
IM	intramuscular
INH	inhalation
IPPB	intermittent positive pressure breathing
I&O	intake and output
IU	international unit
IUD	intrauterine contraceptive device
IV	intravenous

IVAC	IV controller
IVP	intravenous pyelogram
IVPB	IV piggyback
K	potassium
Kg	kilogram
L	left
L	liter
lat.	lateral
lb	pound
LH	luteinizing hormone
liq	liquid
LLQ	left lower quadrant
LMP	last menstrual period
LR	lactated Ringer's
LUQ	left upper quadrant
M	meter
m	minum
m2	meter squared
m3	cubic meter
MCA	motorcycle accident
mcg	microgram
mEq	milliequivalent
MI	myocardial infraction
mg	milligram
min	minute
mixt	mixture
ml	milliliter
mm	millimeter
mo	month
mol	mole
MVA	motor vehicle accident

Na	sodium
NC	nasal cannula
neg	negative
ng	nonogram
NKA	no known allergies
noc	night
NPO	nothing by mouth (nothing per os)
NV	neurovascular
O2	oxygen
OD	right eye
OOB	out of bed
OR	operating room
ORIF	open reduction, internal fixation
OS	left eye
os	mouth
OTC	over the counter
OU	each eye
oz	ounce
p	after
P	pulse
P56	plasmalyte 56
PaCO2	arterial cardon dioxide tension (pressure)
PaO2	arterial oxygen tension (pressure)
PCN	penicillin
PEEP	post end expiratory pressure
PERRLA	pupils equal, round & reactive to light & accommodation
pH	hydrogen ion concentration
po	by mouth
PE	physical examination
post/op	postoperatively

prep	preparation
pre op	preoperatively
prn	as needed
PT	patient
q	every
qAM	every morning
qd	everyday
qh	every hour
QID	four times a day
QOD	every other day
qPM	every night
q2h	every 2 hours
q3h	every 3 hours
q4h	every 4 hours
q6h	every 6 hours
q12h	every 12 hours
qs	quantity sufficient
qt	quart
R	respirations
r	right
RBC(s)	red blood count or cell(s)
REM	rapid eye movement
RLQ	right lower quadrant
R/O	rule out
ROM	range of motion
RUQ	right upper quadrant
Rx	therapy, treatment or prescription
s	without
SQ or SC	subcutaneous
Sig	label
SIMV	synchronized intermittent mandatory ventilation

SL	sublingual
sol	solution
ss	one half
Stat	at once
SOB	short of breath
surg	surgical
Sxs	symptoms
supp	suppository
syr	syrup
T	temperature
T&A	tonsillectomy & adenoidectomy
Tab	tablet
TAH	total abdominal hysterectomy
tbsp	tablespoon
temp	temperature
TID	three times daily
TPR	temperature, pulse, respirations
Top	topical
Tinc	tincture
tsp	teaspoon
U	unit
UA	urinalysis
UV	ultraviolet
vag	vaginal
VD	venereal disease
VO	verbal order
vol	volume
VS	vital signs
WBC	white blood count
wk	week
WNL	within normal limits

wt	weight
yr	year
>	greater than
<	less than
=	equal
≠	not equal
2°	secondary degree
%	precent
@	at

MEASUREMENT EQUIVALENTS

METRIC SYSTEM

1 liter (L) = 1,000 milliliters (ml)
1 L. = 1,000 cubic centimeters (cc)
1 grain (gr) = 60 milligrams (mg)
1 gram (G) = 1,000 mg
1 mg = 1,000 micrograms (mcg)
1 cc = 1 ml
1 ounce (oz) = 30 G
1 ml = 16 minims (m)
1 mcg = 0.001 mg
1 kilogram (kg) = 1,000 G
1 kg = 2.2 pounds (lbs)
2.5 centimeters (cm) = 1 inch (in)
1 G = 1,000 kg
15 gr = 1 G

APOTHECARY

60 grains (gr) = 1 dram
8 drams = 1 ounce
16 ounces = 1 pint (pt)
60 minims = 1 dram
480 minims = 1 ounce
1 dram = 1 teaspoon (tsp)
4 drams = 1 tablespoon (tbls)
30 ml = 1 oz.

HOUSEHOLD

8 oz = 1 cup
1 teaspoon = 5 ml
1 glass = 240 ml
2 tablespoons = 1 oz
1 pint = 500 ml
1 quart (qt) = 1000 ml
1 minim = 1 drop (gtt)
1 oz = 30 ml
1 pound = 16 oz
1 gallon = 4 quarts
1 quart = 2 pints

24 HOUR CLOCK

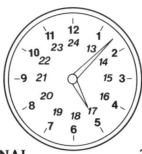

CONVENTIONAL 12 HOUR TIME	24 HOUR CLOCK TIME
12:01 AM	0001
1:00 AM	0100
1:30 AM	0130
2:00 AM	0200
3:00 AM	0300
4:00 AM	0400
5:00 AM	0500
6:00 AM	0600
7:00 AM	0700
8:00 AM	0800
9:00 AM	0900
10:00 AM	1000
11:00 AM	1100
12 noon	1200
1:00 PM	1300
2:00 PM	1400
3:00 PM	1500
4:00 PM	1600
5:00 PM	1700
6:00 PM	1800
7:00 PM	1900
8:00 PM	2000
9:00 PM	2100
10:00 PM	2200
11:00 PM	2300
12 midnight	2400

NORMAL LABORATORY VALUES

This section includes normal values for laboratory tests most likely to be used in the hospital, clinic, or home health care setting. Because most laboratory studies are reported in SI (International System of Measurement) units, they are included when appropriate.

ACID PHOSPHATE (ACP)

Adult: 0.10-0.8 U/ml (Bessey-Lowry)
              1.0-4.0 U/ml (King-Armstrong)
              0.5-2.0 U/ml (Bodansky)
              0.056 U/ml (Roy)
              0.1-2.0 U/ml (Gutman-Gutman)
              0.0-1.0 U/L at 37 C (SI units)
Child: 6.4-15.2 U/ml; not usually done on children

ALANINE AMINOTRANSFERASE (ALT)
Formerly Serum Glutamic-Oxaoacetic Transaminase

4-35 U/L at 37 C (SI units)
5-49 Sigma Frankel U/ml
5-40 IU/L
Values may be lower in women.

ALKALINE PHOSPHATASE (ALP)

Adult: 4-12 units/100 ml   (King-Armstrong)
              1.5-4.5 U/100 ml (Bodansky)
              0.8-2.3 units/100 ml   (Bessey-Lowry)
              25-92 U/L at 30 C (SI units)
Child: Less than 2 yrs 85-235 ImU/ml
              2-8 yrs: 65-210 ImU/mL
              9-15 yrs: 60-300 ImU/ml (active bone growth)
              16-21 yrs: 30-200 ImU/ml
Normal values for children will depend on bone growth only.

AMYLASE
(Serum Amylase, Urine Amylase)

Adult:	Serum:	56-190 IU/L
		110-300 U/L (SI units)
	Urine:	6.5-48 IU/hr. (varies)
		6.5 to 48 U/L (SI units)

Child: Normal values would be the same with correction for size

ARTERIAL BLOOD GASES (ABGs)

Adult:	pH:	.35-7.44 (SI units)
	pO2:	80-100 mmHg
		12.64 to 13.30 kPaa (SI units)
	pCO2:	35-45 mmHg
		4.66-5.32 kPaa (SI units)
	HCO3:	22-26 mEq/L
		22-26 mmol/L (SI units)
	BE:	+2 to -2
		+2 to -2 mmol/L (SI units)
Child:	pH:	7.36-7.44

Other values are similar to adult

ASPARTATE AMINOTRANSFERASE (AST)
Formerly Serum Glutamtic-Pyruvic Transaminase

5-35 IU/L
10-35 U/L at 37 C (SI units)

BILIRUBIN/ICTERUS INDEX (BLOOD)

Direct:	Adult:	0.1-0.3 mg/100 ml
		1.7-5.0 mmol/L (SI units)
	Newborn:	0.1-0.8 mg/100 ml
		1.7-5.0 mmol/L (SI units)
Indirect:	Adult:	0.2-0.8 mg/200 ml
		1.7-17 mmol/L (SI units)
	Newborn:	1-11 mg/100 ml

Icterus Index: 4-6U

Total: Adult: 0.1-1.0 mg/100 ml
                           1.7-20 mmol/L (SI units)
                Child: 2.0-0.8 mg/100 ml
                Newborn:1.0-12.0 mg/100 ml
                           17-205 mmol/L (SI units)

BLEEDING TIME

Adult and Child:
    1-6 minutes for bleeding to stop (Ivy: forearm)
    1-3 minutes for bleeding to stop (Duke: earlobe)
Newborn:
    1-5 mintues for bleeding to stop (Ivy)

BLOOD UREA NITROGEN (BUN)

Man: 10-25 mg/100 ml
Woman: 8-20 mg/100 ml
Child: 8-18 mg/100 ml
Newborn: 5-15 mg/100 ml

CHOLESTEROL

Adult: Less than 200 mg/100 ml
                3.9-6.5 mmol/liter (SI units)
Child: 5-100 mg/100 ml

CLOTTING TIME
(COAGULATION TIME) (LEE-WHITE)

Adult and child: 5-15 minutes

COAGULATION FACTOR CONCENTRATION TEST

I-Fibrinogen: 60-100 mg/ml
II-Prothrombin: 10-15 concentration
III-Tissue thromboplastin
IV-Calcium
V-Proaccelerin: 5%-10% concentration
VII-Proconcetrin: 5%-20% concentration

VIII-Antigemophilic globulin: 30%-35% concentration
IX-Thromboplastin: 30% concentration
X-Stuart-Prower: 8%-10% concentration
XI-Morphilic: 20%-30% concentration
XII-Hageman: 0%
XIII-Fibrin-stabilizing: 1% concentration

COMPLETE BLOOD COUNT (CBC)

RBC:
Adult:
Men: 4.7-6.1 million/mm3
               4.7 to 6.1 x 1012/L (SI units)
Women: 4.2-5.4 million/mm3
               4.2-5.4 x 1012/L (SI units)
Infants and child: 3.8-5.5 million
               3.8-5.5 x 1012/L (SI units)
Newborns: 4.8-7.1 million
               4.8-7.1 x 1012/L (SI units)

RBC indices:
MCV: 80-95 mm3
               80-95 fl (SI units)
Newborns: 96-108 mm3
               96-108 fl (SI units)

MCHC: 32%-36% or g/100 ml
               0.32-0.36 conc. frac. (SI units)
Newborns: 2-33g
               0.32-0.33 conc. frac. (SI units)

MCH: 27-31 pg (SI units)
Newborns: 2-24 pg (SI units)

HCT:
Adult: 42%-52% (male)
               0.42-0.54 vol. frac. (SI units)
               37-47 (female) (pregnancy greater than 33%)
               0.37-0.47 vol. frac. (SI units)

Child:	31-43%
	0.31-0.43 vol. frac. (SI units)
Infant:	30-40%
	0.30-0.40 vol. frac. (SI units)
Newborn:	44-64%
	0.44-0.64 vol. frac. (SI units)

HGB:
Adult:	14-18 g/100ml (male)
	2.09-2.79 mmol/L (SI units)
	12-16 g/100 ml (female) (pregnancy less than 11G)
	1.86-2.48 mmol/L (SI units)
Child:	11-16 g/100 ml
Infant:	10-15 g/100 ml
Newborn:	14-24 g/100 ml

Platelets:
Adult:	1500-400 thousand cu mm
	0.15-0.4 x 1012/L (SI units)
Child:	Same
Newborn:	150 thousand cu mm
	0.15 x 1012/L (SI units)

WBC:
Adult:	5-10 thousand cu mm
	5-11 x 109/L (SI units)
Child less	6.2-17 thousand cu mm
than 2 yrs.	6.2-17 x 109/L (SI units)
Newborn:	9-30 thousand cu mm

DIFF WBC (Adult and Child)

Neutrophils:	3-7 thousand or 55%-70%
	0.55-0.70 mean frac. (SI units)
Eosinophils:	50-400 or 2%-7%
	0.027 mean frac. (SI units)
Basophils:	25-100 or .5-1%
	0.003 mean frac. (SI units)

Lymphocytes: 1-4 thousand or 20%-40%
                 0.34 mean frac. (SI units)
Monocytes: 100-600 or 2%-8%
                 0.04 mean frac. (SI units)

CREATININE

Adult: 0.6-1.3 mg/100ml
           53-100 mmol/L (SI units)
Child: 0.4-1.2 mg/100ml

CREATININE CLEARANCE (24 hour URINE)

Adult: 40-140 ml/min (male)
           0.2-0.3 mmol/kg/24 hrs (SI units)
           85 to 125 ml/min (female)
           0.1-0.2 mmol/kg/24 hrs (SI units)
Child: 98-150 ml/min (male)
Child: 95-123 ml/min (female)

ELECTROLYTES (ELECTROLYTE PANEL)

CO_2:   24-30 mEq/L
Chloride:
Adult: 90-110 mEq/L
           95-105 mmol/L (SI units)
Child: 101-105 mEq/L
Newborn: 93-112 mEq/L
Potassium:
Older Adult: 3.5-5.0 mEq/L
Adult: 3.5-5.5 mEq/L
           3.5-5.5 mmol/L (SI units)
Child: 3.5-4.7 mEq/L
Newborn: .0-7.7 mEq/L
Sodium:
Older Adult: 136-145 mEq/L
Adult: 136-145 mEq/L
           136-145 mmol/L (SI units)
Child: 138-145 mEq/L

Newborn: 126-166 mEq/L
Calcium:
Adult: 9-10.5 mg/100 ml
               2-3 mmol/L (SI units)
Child: 3.9-4.6 mg/ionized
Magnesium:
Adult: 1.6-3.0 mEq/L
               0.7-1.1 mmol/L (SI units)
Child: 1.7-2.2 mEq/L
Phosphorus:
Adult: 2.5-4.5 mg/100 ml
               0.8-1.5 mmol/L (SI units)
Child: 3.5-5.8 mg/100 ml
Newborn: 2.4-5.9 mEq/L
Bicarbonate: 29 mEq/L
Proteinate: 15 mEq/L
Organic acids: 3 mEq/L
Sulfate: 1 mEq/L

ELECTROPHORESIS

Hemoglobin:
   HgA1:   95%-98%
   HgA2:   2%-3%
   HgF: 0.8%-2%
   Hgbs: 0%
   Hgbc: 0%
Serum:
   Albumin   3.3-4.5 g/100 ml
                     33-45 g/L (SI units)
   A2-Globulin   0.5-1.0 g/100ml
                     5-10 g/L (SI units)
   Beta-Globulin   0.7-1.2g/100ml
                     7-12 g/L (SI units)
   Gamma Globulin   0.5-1.6 gm/100ml
                     5-16 g/L (SI units)
Urine: 1/3 of total protein is albumin

GLUCOSE/SUGAR (URINE)

Random urine: Negative
24-hr urine: 0.5-1.5 g/24 hrs. (SI units)
Clintest: Negative
Clinistix/Labstix: No color change

GLUCOSE TOLERANCE TEST (GTT)

Fasting: 70-115 mg/100 ml
                3.85-6.05 mmol/L (SI units)
30 min less than 200 mg/100ml
                1.65-3.30 mmol/L (SI units)
1 hr less than 200 mg/100 ml
                1.10-2.75 mmol/L (SI units)
2 hr less than 140 mg/100 ml
                0.28-0.83 mmol/L (SI units)
3 hr 70-115 mg/100 ml
                3.85-6.05 mmol/L (SI units)
Urine: Negative for all urine

IMMUNOGLOBULINS (IG)

IgA: 85-385 mg/100 ml
              1.1-5.6 g/L (SI units)
IgG: 565-1765 mg/100 ml
              8-18 g/L (SI units)
IgM: 55-375 mg/100 ml
              0.54-2.2 g/L (SI units)
IgD: 0.5-3 mg/100 ml
              5-30 mg/L (SI units)
IgE: 0.01-0.04 mg/100 ml
              0.1-0.4 mg/L (SI units)
Newborn: A and M low but will reach adult level by
              puberty. G decreases rapidly for 6 weeks
              and then increases to reach adult level by
              puberty.

ISOENZYMES

Adult:
LDH1:	17%-27%
	0.17-0.27 frac. total (SI units)
LDH2:	28%-38%
	0.28-0.38 frac. total (SI units)
LDH3:	19%-27%
	0.19-0.27 frac. total (SI units)
LDH4:	5%-16%
	0.5 to 0.16 frac. total (SI units)
LDH5:	6%-16%
	0.5-0.16 frac. total (SI units)
Child:	Not done on children.

LACTIC ACID DEHYDROGENASE (LDH)

80-120 Wacker units
120-130 IU/L
150-450 Wroblewski units
90-200 ImU/ml
38-62 U/L at 30 degrees C (SI units)

LUMBAR PUNCTURE (SPINAL TAP)

Color:	Clear
Cell count:	0-8 cu mm
	0-8 x 106/L (SI units)
Protein:	15-45 mg/dl
	150-450 mg/L (SI units)
Pressure:	Less than 200 mm H2O
Chloride:	118-132 mEq/L
	118-132 mmol/L (SI units)
Glucose:	50-75 mg/dl
	2.75-4.40 mmol/L (SI units)

RBC = 0
Lymphocytes: less than 5/mm3

PARTIAL THROMBOPLASTIN TIME (PPT, ACTIVATED PARTIAL THROMBOPLASTIN, APPT)

PTT: 30-45 seconds
APTT: 30-40 seconds

PHENYLKETONURIA IN BLOOD AND URINE (PKU)

Urine: Negative; no color change
Blood Newborn: 1.2-3.5 mg/dl
                   0.07-0.21 mmol/L (SI units)

POSTPRANDIAL BLOOD SUGAR (GLUCOSE TEST) (2-HR POSTPRANDIAL BLOOD SUGAR, 2-HR PPBS OR 2-HR PPG)

Serum: less than 140
Whole blood: less than 120

PROTHROMBIN TIME (PT, PRO-TIME)

11.0-12.5 seconds or 100%

PULMONARY FUNCTION TEST

Total lung capacity: 5500 ml
Vital capacity: 4000-4800 ml
Residual volume: 1200-1500 ml
Expiratory reserve: 1200-1500 ml
Forced vital capacity: 4800 ml
Inspiratory capacity: 2500-3600 ml
Normal values for PFT are predicted for each patient
based on height, weight, and sex.

SEDIMENTATION RATE (SED RATE, ESR)

Men: less than 50 yrs: less than 15 mm/hr (SI units)
Men: greater than 50 yrs: less than 20 mm/hr (SI units)

Women: less than 50 yrs: less than 20 mm/hr (SI units)
Women: greater than 50 yrs: less than 30 mm/hr (SI units)
Children: less than 10 mm/hr (SI Units)

THROMBIN CLOTTING TIME

10-20 seconds

TRIGLYCERIDES (LIPIDS)

Adult: 40-150 mg/100 ml
                0.10-2.10 mmol/L (SI units)
Older adult: 20-200 mg/100 ml

URIC ACID

Serum
Male: 4.0-8.5 mg/dl
            0.24-0.5 mmol/L (SI units)
Female: 2.7-7.3 mg/dl
            0.16-0.43 mmol/L (SI units)
Child: 2.5-5.5 mg/dl
Urine
Adult: 250-750 mg/24 hrs.
            1.48-4.43 mmol/24 hrs. (SI units)
Child: Similar to adult

URINALYSIS, ROUTINE

Specific Gravity (1.005-1.030)
Appearance: Amber yellow, clear
Glucose: Negative
Blood: Negative
Ketones: Negative
Protein: Up to 8mg/dl (Albumin)
Bile: Negative
Bilirubin: Negative
Casts: Occasional hyaline
RBC: Up to 2
Crystals: Negative

WBC:	Negative
Ph:	4.6-8.0 (6.0 avg.)
Odor:	Aromatic

UROBILINOGEN (URINE)

2 hrs:	0.3-1.0 Ehrlich units/dl
24 hrs:	0.05-2.5 mg/24 hrs.
	0.5-4.0 Ehrlich units/24 hrs.
	0.1 to 4.23 micromol/24 hrs. (SI units)

COMMUNICABLE DISEASES

AMEBIASIS

INFECTIVE ORGANISM: *Entamoeba histolytica*

INFECTIOUS SOURCES: Contaminated water and food

METHOD OF SPREAD: Patients and carriers; fecal-oral route

INCUBATION PERIOD: Variable

ACQUIRED IMMUNE DEFICIENCY SYNDROME

INFECTIVE ORGANISM: Human immunodeficiency virus (HIV)

INFECTIOUS SOURCES: Human case

METHOD OF SPREAD: Sexual intercourse, contaminated blood or needles

INCUBATION PERIOD: Up to 10 years, average 2-5 years

ANTHRAX

INFECTIVE ORGANISM: *Bacillus anthracis*

INFECTIOUS SOURCES: Cattle, sheep, horses, goats

METHOD OF SPREAD: Animal hair, hides, waste

INCUBATION PERIOD: Variable

BACILLIARY DYSENTERY (Shigellosis)

INFECTIVE ORGANISM: *Shigella* organisms

INFECTIOUS SOURCES: Contaminated water and food

METHOD OF SPREAD: Patients and carriers; fecal-oral route

INCUBATION PERIOD: 1-4 days

BRUCELLOSIS

INFECTIVE ORGANISM: *Brucella melitensis* and related organisms

INFECTIOUS SOURCES: Milk, meat, tissues, absorbed fetuses and placenta from infected cattle, goats, horses, pigs, blood

METHOD OF SPREAD: Ingestion of or contact with infective material

INCUBATION PERIOD: Average 2 weeks

CHANCROID
INFECTIVE ORGANISM: *Hemophilus ducreyi*
INFECTIOUS SOURCES: Human cases and carriers
METHOD OF SPREAD: Direct sexual contact
INCUBATION PERIOD: 3-5 days

CHICKENPOX (VARICELLA)
INFECTIVE ORGANISM: *Varicella zoster* virus
INFECTIOUS SOURCES: Human cases
METHOD OF SPREAD: Probably respiratory droplets, direct contact, contaminated objects
INCUBATION PERIOD: 13-17 days

DIPHTHERIA
INFECTIVE ORGANISM: *Corynebacterium diphtheriae*
INFECTIOUS SOURCES: Human cases, fomites, raw milk
METHOD OF SPREAD: Nasal and oral secretions, respiratory droplets, direct contact
INCUBATION PERIOD: 2-5 days

ENCEPHALITIS, EPIDEMIC (EASTERN AND WESTERN EQUINE)
INFECTIVE ORGANISM: Viruses
INFECTIOUS SOURCES: Chicken and wild bird mites, horses, hibernating garter snakes
METHOD OF SPREAD: Mosquitoes
INCUBATION PERIOD: Variable

GONORRHEA
INFECTIVE ORGANISM: *Neisseria gonorrhoeae*
INFECTIOUS SOURCES: Urethral and vaginal secretion
METHOD OF SPREAD: Sexual activity
INCUBATION PERIOD: 2-14 days in men and 7-21 days in women

GRANULOMA INGUINALE
INFECTIVE ORGANISM: *Donovania granulomatis*
INFECTIOUS SOURCES: Infectious exudate
METHOD OF SPREAD: Sexual intercourse
INCUBATION PERIOD: Unknown; varies 1-23 weeks

HEPATITIS A
INFECTIVE ORGANISM: Hepatitis A virus
INFECTIOUS SOURCES: Person-to-person contact,
contaminated food or water; feces; blood; urine
METHOD OF SPREAD: Fecal-oral route, ingestion of/or
partial inoculation with infected blood or blood products
INCUBATION PERIOD: 2-6 weeks

HEPATITIS B
INFECTIVE ORGANISM: Hepatitis B virus
INFECTIOUS SOURCES: Infected blood donor; contaminated
injection equipment
METHOD OF SPREAD: Parental injection of human blood,
plasma, thrombin, fibrinogen, packed cells, and other blood
products from an infected person; contaminated needles and
syringes; venereal contact
INCUBATION PERIOD: 4-25 weeks

INFLUENZA (GRIP, FLU)
INFECTIVE ORGANISM: Virus (types A and B) Myxoviruses
INFECTIOUS SOURCES: Human cases, animal reservoir
METHOD OF SPREAD: Respiratory
INCUBATION PERIOD: 48 hours

LASSA FEVER
INFECTIVE ORGANISM: Lassa virus
INFECTIOUS SOURCES: Rats
METHOD OF SPREAD: Unknown
INCUBATION PERIOD: Unknown

LYMPHOGRANULOMA VENEREUM

INFECTIVE ORGANISM: *Chlamydia trachomatis*

INFECTIOUS SOURCES: Human cases

METHOD OF SPREAD: Sexual intercourse, indirect contact with contaminated articles or clothing

INCUBATION PERIOD: 7-28 days

MALARIA

INFECTIVE ORGANISM: *Plasmodium vivax, P. falciparum, P. malariae and P. ovale*

INFECTIOUS SOURCES: Human cases

METHOD OF SPREAD: Female anopheles mosquitoes

INCUBATION PERIOD: Variable, depending on strain 10-35 days average

MARBURG VIRUS DISEASE

INEFFECTIVE ORGANISM: Virus

INFECTIOUS SOURCES: Africian green monkey

METHOD OF SPREAD: Tissues, and cell cultures

INCUBATION PERIOD: Variable

MEASLES (RUBEOLA)

INFECTIVE ORGANISM: Paramyxovirus

INFECTIOUS SOURCES: Human cases

METHOD OF SPREAD: Nasopharyngeal secretions, blood, urine

INCUBATION PERIOD: 10-20 days

MENINGITIS ACUTE BACTERIAL

INFECTIVE ORGANISM: *Neisseria meningitidis*

INFECTIOUS SOURCES: Human cases and carriers

METHOD OF SPREAD: Respiratory droplets

INCUBATION PERIOD: 2-10 days

MONONUCLEOSIS, Infectious
INFECTIVE ORGANISM: Epstein-Barr virus
INFECTIOUS SOURCES: Human cases and carriers
METHOD OF SPREAD: Probably oral-pharyngeal route, blood transfusions in susceptible recipients
INCUBATION PERIOD: 4-7 weeks

MUMPS
INFECTIVE ORGANISM: Virus
INFECTIOUS SOURCES: Human cases (early)
METHOD OF SPREAD: Respiratory droplets, direct contact
INCUBATION PERIOD: 14-21 days

PARATYPHOID FEVER
INFECTIVE ORGANISM: *Salmonella paratyphi A* and *B* and related organisms
INFECTIOUS SOURCES: Contaminated food, milk, water; rectal tubes; barium enemas
METHOD OF SPREAD: Infected urine and feces
INCUBATION PERIOD: 3-25 days

PNEUMOCOCCAL PNEUMONIA
INFECTIVE ORGANISM: *Streptococcus pneumoniae*
INFECTIOUS SOURCES: Human carriers; patient's own pharynx
METHOD OF SPREAD: Respiratory droplets
INCUBATION PERIOD: Variable

PNEUMONIC PLAGUE
INFECTIVE OREGANISM: *Yersinia pestis*
INFECTIOUS SOURCES: Human carriers
METHOD OF SPREAD: Respiratory droplets
INCUBATION PERIOD: Variable

POLIOMYELITIS
INFECTIVE ORGANISM: Polioviruses (Types I, II, III)
INFECTIOUS SOURCES: Human cases and carriers
METHOD OF SPREAD: Infected feces, pharyngeal secretions
INCUBATION PERIOD: 7-14 days

RABIES
INFECTIVE ORGANISM: Virus
INFECTIOUS SOURCES: Infected bats, skunks, foxes, raccoons, dogs, cats and cattle
METHOD OF SPREAD: Bite of rabid animal
INCUBATION PERIOD: Average 4-6 wks.

ROCKY MOUNTAIN SPOTTED FEVER (TICK FEVER)
INFECTIVE ORGANISM: *Rickettsia rickettsii*
INFECTIOUS SOURCES: Infected wild rodents, dogs, wood ticks, dog ticks
METHOD OF SPREAD: Tick bites
INCUBATION PERIOD: 3-10 days; 7 days average

RUBELLA (GERMAN MEASLES)
INFECTIVE ORGANISM: Virus
INFECTIOUS SOURCES: Human cases
METHOD OF SPREAD: Nasopharyngeal secretions, feces or urine
INCUBATION PERIOD: 14-21 days

SCARLET FEVER
INFECTIVE ORGANISM: *Steptococcus hemolyticus*, group A *B-hemolytic streptocci*
INFECTIOUS SOURCES: Human cases; infected foods
METHOD OF SPREAD: Nasal and oral secretion, ingestion of contaminated food, milk, direct contact
INCUBATION PERIOD: 2-4 days

SYPHILIS
INFECTIVE ORGANISM: *Treponema pallidum*
INFECTIOUS SOURCES: Infected exudate of blood
METHOD OF SPREAD: Sexual activity; contact with open lesions; blood transfusions transplacenta inoculation
INCUBATION PERIOD: 1-13 weeks, usually 3-4 weeks

TETANUS (LOCKJAW)
INFECTIVE ORGANISM: *Clostridium tetani*
INFECTIOUS SOURCES: Contaminated soil
METHOD OF SPREAD: Horses and cattle feces
INCUBATION PERIOD: 5-10 days

TRICHINOSIS
INFECTIVE ORGANISM: *Trichinella spiralis*
INFECTIOUS SOURCES: Infected pigs
METHOD OF SPREAD: Ingestion of infected pork that is uncooked
INCUBATION PERIOD: 2-28 days

TUBERCULOSIS
INFECTIVE ORGANISM: *Mycobaterium tuberculosis*
INFECTIOUS SOURCES: Sputum or droplets from human cases; milk from infected cows (rare U.S.)
METHOD OF SPREAD: Sputum; respiratory droplets, direct contact
INCUBATION PERIOD: About 4-6 weeks

TULAREMIA (RABBITE or DEER-FLY FEVER)
INFECTIVE ORGANISM: *Pasteurella tularensis* (Francissela tularensis)
INFECTIOUS SOURCES: Wild rodents and rabbits
METHOD OF SPREAD: Handling infected wild animals; ingestion of undercooked infected meat; drinking contaminated water; bites from infected flies, ticks

INCUBATION PERIOD: 1-10 days

TYPHOID FEVER
INFECTIVE ORGANISM: *Salmonella typhi*
INFECTIOUS SOURCES: Contaminated food and water
METHOD OF SPREAD: Infected urine and feces
INCUBATION PERIOD: 3-25 days

TYPHUS, EPIDEMIC (JAIL FEVER)
INFECTIVE ORGANISM: *Rickettsia typhi* (mooseri)
INFECTIOUS SOURCES: Infected rodents
METHOD OF SPREAD: Flea bites
INCUBATION PERIOD: 7-14 days

WHOOPING COUGH (PERTUSSIS)
INFECTIVE ORGANISM: *Bordetella pertussis*
INFECTIOUS SOURCES: Human cases
METHOD OF SPREAD: Infected bronchial secretions
INCUBATION PERIOD: 5-21 days, usually 10 days

DRUG

ADMINISTRATION

DRUG ADMINISTRATION

Table of Contents

COMMON DRUGS

ANABOLIC STEROIDS

ACTIONS: Promotes anabolic processes leading to increased body tissue, increased bone development and overall weight gain. Stimulates erythropoiesis.

USES: Weight gain, adjunctive therapy for tissue depleating conditions, osteoporosis, refractory anemias.   Additionally used to combat catabolic effects of therapy with corticosterioids.   Also used in patients suffering prolonged immobilization.

GENERAL COMMENTS: Anabolic steroids reverse catabolic reactions, multiple adverse androgenic problems may arise, to include in females: acne, oily skin, undesirable weight gain, hirsutism, altered libido and hoarseness.   In males; premature epipuyseal closure, acne, priapism and testicular atrophy, gynecomastia and epididymitis may occur. Various GI disturbances occur.   May be hepatoxic.   In females, vaginal abnormalities may include bleeding. Hypercalcemia is possible.

Examples of Drugs in this Classification:

Generic	Trade	Comments
Ethylestrenol	Maxibolin	Available PO. Watch for adverse androgenic effects. Monitor liver function tests. Contraindicated with obstructive prostatic hypertrophy and male breast cancer, or

Generic	Trade	Comments
		prostatic carcinoma, compromised renal or hepatic patients or those with hypercalcemia. Caution should be exercised with therapy in prepubertal males, diabetics, patients taking ACTH, corticosteroids or anticoagulants. Monitor male children under seven years of age for precocious sexual development. Promote diet high in calories and protein. May alter various laboratory values for up to 3 weeks after therapy is discontinued. Assess for signs or symptoms of hypoglycemia.
Nandrolone decanoate	Androlone-D, Deca-Durabolin Hybolin Decanoate	Available IM. Observe closely and report adverse androgenic effects. Monitor liver function tests.

Generic	Trade	Comments
Nandrolone Phenpro-pionate	Anabolin, Anorolone, Hypolin, Improved Nandrobolic	Contraindicated in obstructive prostatic hypertrophy, carcinoma of male breast or prostate, cardiac, renal or hepatic compromised patients. Caution should be exercised with therapy in prepubertal males, diabetics, corticosteroids or anticoagulants. Monitor male children under seven years of age for precocious sexual development. Promote diet high in calories and protein if possible. May alter various laboratory values for up to 3 weeks after therapy is discontinued. Assess for signs or symptoms of hypoglycemia.
Stanozolol	Winstrol	Available PO. Observe and report adverse androgenic effects. Monitor liver function tests. Contraindicated with obstructive prostatic hypertrophy, carcioma of male breast or prostate, cardiac, renal or hepatic

Generic	Trade	Comments
		compromised patients. Caution should be exercised with therapy in prepubertal males, diabetics, patients taking ACTH, corticosteroids or anticoagulants. Monitor male children under seven years of age for precocious sexual development. Promote diet high in calories and protein if possible. May alter various laboratory values for up to 3 weeks after therapy is discontinued. Assess for signs or symptoms of hypoglycemia.

ANALGESICS, NON-NARCOTIC

ACTIONS: Relief of pain by blocking generation of pain impulses through inhibition of prostaglandin synthesis.

USES: Minor pain relief.

GENERAL COMMENTS: For mild to moderate pain. May be used for acute or chronic pain: Toothache, headache, malaise due to viruses, minor injuries, rheumatic joint complaints. These are available in many combinations of aspirin, acetaminophen, and caffeine ingredients. Over-the-counter preparations may be abused. Instruct to take dose as recommended by physician or package directions. Over-the-counter preparations are often involved in childhood poisonings.

Examples of drugs used in this classification:

Generic	Trade	Comments
Acetamino-phen	Tylenol, Tempra, Datril	Non-narcotic analgesic. May be given PO, rectal. Tablets may be crushed. For mild to moderate pain. Avoid use in alcoholics due to hepatotocixity. Also an antipyretic.
Aspirin	ASA, Bayer, Empirin, Ecotrin	Non-narcotic analgesic. May be given PO, rectal. Administer with food, milk or to decrease GI upset may be crushed. Discard tablets if vinegar odor is present. For mild to moderate pain. Prophylactic use to prevent myocardial infarction (1 tablet daily in a.m.). Effective for rheumatic joint diseases, as an antiflammatory. Tinnitus may indicate toxicity. Not recommended for children due to association with Reye's syndrome.
Codeine	Tylenol #3	Administer with milk or food to prevent GI upset. 30 mg codeine=650 mg aspirin (analgesic effect).
Hydromor-phone	Dilaudid	Narcotic analgesic. May be given PO, rectal, SC, IM, IV slow. For moderate to severe pain.

Generic	Trade	Comments
Meperidine	Demerol	Narcotic analgesic. May be given PO, SC, IM, IV slow. For moderate to severe pain.
Morphine sulfate		Narcotic analgesic. May be given PO, rectal, SC, IM, IV slow. Urinary retention may occur, encourage voiding.
Pentazocine	Talwin	Narcotic analgesic. May be given PO, SC, IM, IV. For moderate to severe pain.
Propoxy-phene	Darvon	May be given PO. Narcotic analgesic. Capsules may be opened and mixed with food. For mild to moderate pain. Smoking decreases effectiveness.

ANDROGENS

ACTION: Androgens   act   on   select   tissues   in androgen-deficient males facilitating normal development. In the case of Danazol; FSH and LH are decreased which leads to atropy of endometrial tissue by halting amenorrhea and ovulation.

USES: Endometriosis,   fibrocystic   breast   disease, hypogonadism, impotence in males, postpartum breast engorgement, breast cancer in women, cryptorchidism in males post-puberty.

GENERAL   COMMENTS: In   females   can   cause numerous androgenic reactions such as: acne, weight gain, hirsutism, decrease in breast size, male-pattern baldness, vaginal bleeding, emotional liability and menstrual irregularities. May cause GI upset. In males: acne, priapism, epiphyseal closure (premature), penile enlargement, impotency can occur.

Examples of Drugs in This Classification:

Generic	Trade	Comments
Danazol	Danocrine	Available PO. Can cause thrombocytopenia, dizziness, headache, depression, irritability, hypertension, hematuria. Occasionally muscle cramps can occur. Not used if vaginal bleeding which has been diagnosed is present. If possible, therapy should include high protein/calorie diet. Vaginitis can occur; stress good personal hygiene. When administered for fibrocytic breast disease, encourage frequent breast exam. If mass enlarges during therapy, report immediately. Observe for adrogenic effects closely, some are not reversible. Exercise caution in patients with migraine headaches or seizure disorders.

Generic	Trade	Comments
Fluoxyme-terone	Android-F, Halotestin, Ora-Testryl	Available PO. Vaginitis can occur, stress good personal hygiene. Bladder irritability can occur. Various vaginal irregularities are possible including bleeding. Contraindicated in males with obstructive prostatic hypertrophy, breast cancer, prostatic cancer. Caution should be exercised with therapy in patients with impaired cardiac, renal or hepatic status. Monitor closely when patient is on ACTH therapy, cortico-steroids or anticoagulants. Hypercalcemia can occur. Observe closely for androgenic side effects in female, some may not be reversible. Generalized edema may be observed. May cause hypoglycemia.
Testosterone	Depotest Testa-c Everone	Available IM. Observe closely for and report adverse androgenic effects. Possible masculization of female infants, therefore contraindicated in women who may become pregnant. Further contraindications: prostatic hypertrophy with obstruction, CHF, renal or

Generic	Trade	Comments
		hepatic compromise. Can lead to hypoglycemia. In males discontinue use if priapism or gynecomastia occur. Inject deep IM. Affects various laboratory results for up to 3 weeks after therapy is discontinued.

ANTACIDS

ACTIONS: Neutralize acid in the stomach.

USES: For use in conditions with excess production of hydrochloric acid as in gastric or peptic ulcers, hiatal hernia, esophageal reflex and gastritis.

GENERAL COMMENTS: Administer between meals unless otherwise noted. Tablets should be chewed throughly and liquids shaken well. Liquid preparations are reported to be more effective than tablets. Encourage increased fluid intake when taking antacids. Assess for pattern of stools for constipation or diarrhea as both are common side effects. Do not administer antacids within 1-2 hours of other drugs to prevent interactions.

Examples of Drugs in This Classification:

Generic	Trade	Comments
ALUMINUM ANTACIDS		
Aluminum carbonate	Basaljel	May be given PO. Major side effect is constipation. Administer 1 hour after meals/bedtime.

Generic	Trade	Comments
Aluminum hydroxide	AlternaGEL Alu-Cap Alu-Tab Amphojel Dialume	May be given PO, intragastric drip. Impaction or intestinal obstruction may occur with use, monitor stools.
Aluminum phosphate	Phosphaljel	Monitor serum phosphate levels and report elevation.

CALCIUM CARBONATES

Calcium carbonate	Alka-mints Titralac, Tums	May be given PO: Tablets or powder. Acid rebound with gastric hypersecretion may occur with chronic use. Discourage long term dependence. Monitor stools for constipation. Assess for hypercalcemia with nausea, vomiting, thrist, dry mouth, constipation, fatigue, muscle weakness, joint pain.

MAGNESIUM ANTACIDS

Magnesium carbonate Magnesium oxide	Mag-Ox 400 Uro-Mag Maox	May be given PO. Laxative effect, monitor for diarrhea. May be given PO. Laxative effect.
Magnesium Salt	Milk of Magnesia	Give before meals/bedtime. Laxative effect.

Generic	Trade	Comments

ALUMINUM & MAGNESIUM COMBINATIONS:

	Maalox	Side effects from either
	Aludrox	category may occur.
	Mylanta	
	Gelusil	
	Di-Gel	

ANTIANXIETY AGENTS

ACTION: These agents act at the limbic and subcortical levels of the brain to depress the CNS.

USES: Treatment of anxiety and tension, acute alcohol withdrawal and in some cases an adjunctive therapy in epilepsy.

GENERAL COMMENTS: Generally these drugs may cause drowsiness, occasionally confusion, transient hypotension and GI discomfort. Dry mouth is common. Substance abuse and addiction are possible. Psychomotor skills are usually impaired to some degree. Blurred vision has been reported. Cimetidine may increase sedative effect. Dosage should be reduced in debilitated or elderly patients. Antianxiety agents should never be combined with alcohol. These drugs are not for everyday stress of living. Contraindicated in anxiety-free psychiatric disorders.

Examples of Drugs in This Classification:

Generic	Trade	Comments
Alprazolam	Xanax	Available PO. Not administered if acute narrow-angle glaucoma present. Withdraw therapy gradually, withdrawal

Generic	Trade	Comments
		symptoms may occur. Not for long-term therapy (greater than 4 months). May be therapeutic in depression. Controlled substance schedule IV.
Buspirone HCl	BuSpar	Available PO. Method of action undetermined. No reported drug interaction. Generally less sedating than other drugs in this class. Not as effective as an anticonvulsant or muscle relaxant. Take with food. Desired effects usually observed after 3-4 weeks of therapy. No demonstrated abuse qualities. Not a controlled substance.
Chlordiaze-poxide	Libritabs Librium Lipoxide	Available PO, IM or IV. Use cautiously in patients with blood dyscrasias or concurrent therapy with anticoagulants. Commonly used for alcohol withdrawal. Controlled substance schedule IV.
Diazepam	Valium Valrelease	Available PO, IM, IV. Use as adjunctive therapy in seizure disorders. Used as a skeletal muscle relaxant for acute severe spasm.

Generic	Trade	Comments
		Respiratory depressant, contraindicated in patients with severe pulmonary compromise. With IV use, inject no more than 5 mg./min. Have O_2 and emergency resuscitative equipment at bedside when administering. Preferred drug for status epilepticus. Naloxone does not counteract diazepam-induced respiratory depression. Controlled substance schedule IV.
Hydroxyzine HCl	Atarax Durrax Quiess Vistaril	Available PO or IM. Do not administer in patients who are comatose or in shock. Potentiates other CNS drugs. Used post-operatively as an antiemetic with narcotic analgesics. IM route use Z-Track, never give IV.
Lorazepam	Ativan Loraz	Available PO, IM, or IV. No drug interactions reported. Withdraw therapy slowly, withdrawal symptoms may occur. Shorter half-life than other benzodiazapines. Controlled substance schedule IV.

ANTIARRHYTHMICS

ACTIONS: Reduces electrical irregularity of the heart; to correct arrhythmias.

USES: Abnormal electrical pattern noted on ECG, Holter monitor assessment, possible irregular pulse, complaints of palpitations, weakness, dizziness. Symptoms may occur when stimulants are taken (caffeine, cigarettes, medications) or may occur spontaneously. There may be no noticeable symptoms.

GENERAL COMMENTS: Should be taken exactly as ordered. ECG or Holter monitor is usually ordered prior to start of treatment and periodically to assess treatment effectiveness. Use of over-the-counter drugs should be checked with physician. During IV therapy, close monitoring of vital signs is important, especially the rate and character of the pulse and blood pressure readings.

Examples of Drugs in This Classification:

Generic	Trade	Comments
Amiodarone HCl	Cordarone	Given PO. Used for arrhythmias resistant to other therapy. Use methylcellulose ophthalmic solution in eyes to prevent corneal microdeposits. Monitor B/P, pulse, liver and thyroid tests. Monitor for pulmonary toxicity, chest pain, nonproductive cough, dyspnea.
Atropine sulfate	Atropine	Available IM, IV. Monitor I&O closely, urinary

Generic	Trade	Comments
		retention possible. Assess breath sounds. May be used IM in certain insecticide poisonings. Monitor BP for hypotension. Monitor for arrhythmias.
Bretylium-tosylate	Bretylol	Available IV, IM. Monitor continuous ECG for effectiveness. Monitor BP continuously. Be alert for rebound hypertension 1-2 hours post administration.
Esmolol HCl	Brevibloc	Available IV. Decreases heart rate and blood pressure. Monitor BP closely for hypotension. Must be diluted, do not inject directly. For short-term initial stabilization of heart rate no longer than 48 hours.
Lidocaine	Xylocaine	May be given IV, IM. IV rate must be monitored closely. Continuous ECG monitoring as above. Convulsions may occur with IV use, seizure precautions may be helpful. Serum levels are required, therapeutic is 1.5-6 mcg/ml.

Generic	Trade	Comments
Phenytoin	Dilantin Diphenylen	Also used as anticonvulsant. Tablets may be crushed. May be given PO or IV. Should not be discontinued suddenly. Should be given with food or drink. Caution against alcohol use, which increases drug blood levels. Discontinue if rash appears and notify physician. Balanced diet is important when taking this drug. Regular serum drug levels are required during use, therapeutic is 10-20 mcg/ml.
Procainamide	Procansr Promine Pronestyl Rhythmin	May be given PO, IM, or IV. Tablets may be crushed. May be mixed with food. Monitor temperature for elevation during initial use. IV precautions as above. Regular serum blood levels are required to monitor drug levels. Pulse should be monitored at least daily for duration of treatment and record kept.
Quinidine	Dura-Tabs Quinate Quinidex	May be given PO, IM, or IV. Tablets should not be crushed or chewed.

Generic	Trade	Comments
		Continuous ECG monitoring with IV use and monitor BP for hypotension. Monitor and report the following STAT: QRS complex is prolonged (ECG), no P wave is present (ECG), increase or onset of PVCs (ECG), tachycardia greater than 120, BP drops.
Verapamil	Calan Isoptin	May be given PO, IV. Monitor I & O during initial treatment for renal impairment. Pulse should be taken prior to each dose, irregular rhythms or bradycardia should be reported. Dizziness during initial treatment is common. Use of caffeine products should be limited.

ANTICHOLINERGICS

ACTION: Reduces intestinal mobility and reduce acid production.

USES: For use in conditions with excess intestinal mobility or hydrochloric acid production including peptic ulcers, pylorspasm, irritable colon.

GENERAL COMMENTS: Common side effects include dry mouth, increased heart rate, constipation, blurred vision.

Examples of Drugs in This Classification:

Generic	Trade	Comments
Atropine SO$_4$		May be given PO, SC, IM, IV. Usually given 30 min. before meals. Monitor vital signs, I&O for urinary retention, stools for frequency. Provide mouth care for dryness.
Belladonna	Belladonna Tincture	Given PO. Do not administer with antacid.

ANTICOAGULANTS

ACTIONS: Prevents blood clotting.

USES: Deep vein thrombosis, cerebral vascular accidents or transient ishemic attacks, myocardial infarction, coronary occlusion and coagulation disorders.

GENERAL COMMENTS: Regular evaluation of prothrombin time or other coagulation studies will need to be done to assess the effectiveness of treatment. Assess for bleeding, as these drugs decrease the blood's ability to clot. Bleeding from any body orifice should be reported including: bleeding gums, nosebleeds, blood in urine, feces, saliva and expectorant. The skin should be assessed for bruises and noted. Pressure should be used on all venipuncture sites, cuts, or wounds for a minimum of 5-10 minutes. A medical alert bracelet should be worn by anyone taking these drugs long term. Use of over-the-counter drugs should be checked with physician.

Examples of Drugs in This Classification:

Generic	Trade	Comments
Dicumarol		Available PO. Assess frequently for hemorrhage. Many drug interactions. Monitor prothrombin time. May cause red to orange urine.
Heparin	Caprin Hep Lock	May be given SC, IV. Check label prior to administration for correct dosage. Preferred SC site is the abdomen and using a TB syringe, 25-26 gauge 1/2-5/8 inch needle. Do not aspirate when injecting drug. Do not inject within 2 inches of umbilicus. Apply pressure, but do not massage after injection. Monitor IV heparin closely for correct dose. Antidote is protamine sulfate.
Warfarin Sodium	Coumadin Panwarfin	May be given PO, IV, IM. Tablets may be crushed. Can administer with heparin in same syringe, in emergency. Antidote is vitamin K.

ANTICONVULSANTS

ACTIONS: Prevents convulsive/seizure activity.

USES: Seizures from any cause including seizure disorder, head injury, neural surgery.

GENERAL COMMENTS: Seizure medications are generally prescribed according to the type of seizure activity noted. Drowsiness is a possible side effect in all of the following medications and patients should be cautioned against activities that could be hazardous until exact effect of medication is known. All seizure medications must be taken exactly as ordered. Missed doses may precipitate seizure activity with some medications. Medication should never be discontinued without the approval of the physician, and then it may require several weeks or months to wean the patient off some of these medications. Regular laboratory monitoring is required. All persons taking anticonvulsants should wear a Medic-Alert bracelet at all times. No over-the-counter medications should be taken without consulting the primary health care provider.

Examples of Drugs in This Classification:

Generic	Trade	Comments
Carbamaze-pine	Tegretol	May be given PO. Administer with meals. Therapeutic level 4-12 mcg/ml. Avoid excessive exposure to sunlight due to photosensitivity. Also used in treatment of trigeminal neuralgia, multiple sclerosis.
Clonazepam	Klonopin	May be given PO. Long term use may require dosage adjustment to control seizure activity. Monitor I & O, as drug may affect renal function.

Generic	Trade	Comments
Ethosuximide	Zarontin	May be given PO. Therapeutic level is 40-100 mcg/ml. Store in light-resistant container.
Phenobar- bital	Barbita Luminal	May be given PO, rectal, SC, IM, IV. Tablets may be crushed if mixed with food or drink. Administer IV cautiously, no more than 60 mg/min. Check IV catheter placement prior to administration, extravasa- tion may require skin graft. Physical dependence may occur. Therapeutic level is 10-20 mcg/ml.
Phenytoin	Dilantin	May be given PO, IV. Check suspension strength carefully prior to admin- istration. Shake suspension well. Tablet may be crushed and mixed with food or fluid. Administer with food or fluid. Do not administer IV with any other drug. Flush line with NS before and after IV administra- tion. Therapeutic level is

Generic	Trade	Comments
		10-20 mcg/ml. Assess for jaundice and report if found. Instruct patient in care of teeth and gums as gingival hyperplasia is a common side effect.
Primidone	Mysoline	May be given PO. Tablet may be crushed and mixed with food and drink. Therapeutic level is 5-10 mcg/ml.
Valproic acid	Depakene	May be given PO. Do not crush tablets. Oral solution should not be taken with soft drinks. Therapeutic level is 50-100 mcg/ml.

ANTIDEPRESSANTS

ACTIONS: Allows norepinephrine and or serotonin to accumulate by blocking their reuptake by presynapsic neurons in tricyclic antidepressants. In the case of MAO inhibitors, accumulation of neurotransmitters is accomplished by inhibiting monoamine oxidase.

USES: Treatment of depression.

GENERAL COMMENTS: Sedation, dizziness, headache, blurred vision, orthostatic hypotension, dry mouth, constipation, anorexia, urinary retention, general malaise and confusion have been reported. Contraindicated in recovery phase of MI, prostatic hypertrophy, increases intraocular pressure, or seizure disorders. Exercise caution in patients with urinary retention, cardiovascular disease, thyroid disease or blood dyscrasias. Elderly and debilitated patients require dosage reduction. Inform patient about possible compromise of psychomotor skills. MAO inhibitors are contraindicated with foods containing tryptophan or tyramine. Avoid drinking alcohol while taking these drugs.

Examples of Drugs in This Classification:

Generic	Trade	Comments
Amitriptyline HCl	Amitril Elavil Emitrip Endep Enovil	Adverse drug interactions with MAO inhibitors, epinephrine, norepinephrine, barbiturates, methylphenidate. Chart variations in moods. Monitor for suicidal risk. Assess for urinary retention and constipation. Most sedating tricyclic antidepressant. Requires 10-14 days to achieve initial and therapeutic results. Instruct patient to avoid OTC drugs if possible.
Desipramine HCl	Norpramin Pertofrane	Available PO. Adverse drug interactions with MAO inhibitors, epinephrine, norepinephrine, barbiturates, methylphenidate, cimetidine. Do not withdraw therapy

Generic	Trade	Comments
		suddenly. Orthostatic hypotension not as pronounced as with other tricyclics. Chart variations in mood. Monitor for suicidal risk. Procedures less sedation than other antidepressants. Affects cardiovascular system less. May be prescribed for cardiac patients. Requires 10-14 initial days to achieve therapeutic results.
Doxepin HCl	Adapin Sinequan	Available PO. Possible adverse drug interactions with MAO inhibitors, barbiturates, methylphenidate, cimetidine. Very sedating. Access for urinary retention and constipation. Take at HS. Requires 10-14 days to achieve initial therapeutic results. Well tolerated by geriatric patients.
Fluoxetine HCl	Prozac	Available PO. Reduced anticholinergic adverse effects. May lead to weight loss. Exercise caution in patients with compromised hepatic function. May discontinue abruptly if needed. Give

Generic	Trade	Comments
		doses at AM and at midday. Reduced incidence of GI upset.
Imipramine HCl	Janimine Tipramine Tofranil	Available PO. Possible adverse drug interactions with MAO inhibitors, barbiturates, methylpheidate, cimetidine. Assess for suicidal risk. Assess for urinary retention and constipation. Take at HS. Requires 10-14 days to achieve initial therapeutic results.
Nortriptyline HCl	Aventyl Pamelor	Available PO. Possible adverse drug interactions with MAO inhibitors, barbiturates, methylpheidate, cimetidine. Assess for suicidal risk. Assess for urinary retention and constipation. Take at HS. Requires 10-14 days to achieve initial therapeutic results.
Tranylcy-promine SO4	Parnate	Available PO. MAO inhibitor. Generally not as effective as tricyclics or other antidepressants. Paradoxical hypertension can occur. Adverse drug interactions with amphetamines, ephedrine, levodopa, meperidine,

Generic	Trade	Comments
		methotrimeprazine, methylphenidate, phenylephrine, alcohol, barbiturates, narcotics, dextromethorphan, tricyclic antidepressants. High tyramine ingestion will induce hypertensive crisis. Regitine used to counteract hypertensive crisis. Assess for suicide risk. Provide dietary instruction to avoid foods or beverages, high tyramine or tryptophan. Observe for orthostatic hypotension. Therapeutic results require up to 3 weeks to achieve. Obtain baseline B/P.
Trazodone HCl	Desyrel	Available PO. Possible adverse drug interactions with antihypertensives and MAO inhibitors. Exercise caution in patients with cardiac disease. May cause painful priapism. Assess for suicide risk. Reduced anticholinergic effects & adverse cardiovascular effects. Requires 10-14 days to achieve therapeutic results.

ANTIDIARRHEALS

ACTION: To decrease the fluid volume in and the amount of loose stools.

USES: Frequent loose, watery stools, diarrhea

GENERAL COMMENTS: Encourage fluid intake to prevent dehydration, during episodes of diarrhea, clear liquids should be offered and solid foods avoided, electrolytes should be monitored for imbalances and replaced as needed.

Examples of Drugs in This Classification:

Generic	Trade	Comments
Bismuth subsalicylate	Pepto-Bismol	May be taken PO. Contains large amount of aspirin. Tablets should be chewed or allowed to dissolve before swallowing. Available over-the-counter. Stools may appear black in color.
Kaolin/pectin	Kaopectate	May be taken PO. Available over-the counter.
Loperamide	Imodium	Usually given after each stool up to 16 mg daily. May be given PO. May cause drowsiness/dizziness. Used often for ulcerative colitis. Activated charcoal for overdose.

Generic	Trade	Comment
Diphenosy-late Atropine	Lomotil Lofene	May be given PO. Schedule V drug. Tablets may be crushed.

ANTIHISTAMINES:

ACTION: Blocks the effects of histamine, thereby reducing the edema caused by the release of histamine.

USES: To treat allergies, colds, rhinitis, allergic reactions.

GENERAL COMMENTS: Drowsiness is a common side effect, and the drug may be prescribed for sedation at bedtime. Caution patient against driving or other activities where mental alertness is required. Alcohol and other sedatives should be avoided while taking this medication. Dry mouth and thickened bronchial secretions may occur. Development of tolerance is common over long term use.

Examples of Drugs in This Classification:

Generic	Trade	Comment
Bromphenir-amine	Dimetane Brombay Spentane Veltane	May be given PO, SC, IM, IV. May be taken with food if stomach upset occurs. Notify physician if high fever, chills or mouth ulcers occur.
Dimenhy-drinate	Dramamine Calm-X Dimen Marmine	May be given PO, IM, IV. Used often for motion sickness or as an antiemetic. May be given prior to radiation therapy. Effects last 3-6 hours. May be given purchased over-the-counter.

Generic	Trade	Comment
Diphenhy-drimine	Benadryl Allerdryl Benylin Nordryl Valdrene	May be given PO, IM, IV. Used often for anaphylaxis. May be given as premedication prior to chemotherapy or blood. May be purchased over-the-counter. May be used for sedative effect.
Hydroxyzine HCl	Vistaril Atarax Quiess	May be given PO, IM. Tablets may be crushed. Preferred IM site is deep upper outer quadrant of buttocks.
Promethazine HCl	Methazine Phenergan Pentazine	May be given PO, IM, IV. Tablets may be crushed. May be given as premedication prior to chemotherapy or blood.

ANTIHYPERTENSIVES

ACTION: Lowers the blood pressure (BP).

USES: BP greater 140/90 on three separate occasions. There may be no noticable symptoms or there may be complaints of headaches.

GENERAL COMMENTS: Any blood pressure over 120 diastolic requires immediate medical attention. Where hypertension has been diagnosed blood pressure should be taken in both arms in three positions: lying, sitting and standing.   Non-compliance is a problem with these medications. Medications are used with diet, weight loss and exercise to lower the blood pressure. All patients should be encouraged to discuss side effects with their physician, as

selection of the correct drug for the individual may take some
trial and error.   Missed doses should be taken when
remembered, double doses should not be taken. A medical
alert bracelet is recommended. Blood pressure should be
taken prior to administration of any of these drugs, and drug
held if patient is hypotensive.

DIURETICS, GENERAL COMMENTS: Commonly
known as "water pills," these increase the excretion of urine.
Encourage fluid intake, unless otherwise specified by health
care provider.   Diuretics are usually taken in the a.m.
Weight, intake and output, BUN and creatinine levels should
be monitored during treatment to assess the effectiveness.

Examples of Drugs in This Classification:

Generic	Trade	Comments
Bumetanide	Bumex	May be given PO, IM, IV. Very powerful loop diuretic. Hypokalemia may occur and potassium should be included in diet daily.
Furosemide	Lasix	May be given PO, IM, IV. IV injection should be slow, no faster than 4 mg/min to prevent ototoxicity. Long term exposure to sunlight should be limited, sunscreen should be worn. Potassium levels should be monitored.

Generic	Trade	Comments
Spironolac-tone	Aldactone	May be given PO. Give with food. Tablet may be crushed. Potassium supplementation is not needed with this drug.

BETA BLOCKERS

GENERAL COMMENTS: These medications work by lowering the heart rate, and should be held if pulse is below 60.

Examples of Drugs in This Classification:

Generic	Trade	Comments
Atenolol	Tenormin	Available PO. Assess for hypotension, bradycardia. Therapeutic response achieved after 1-2 weeks. Do not discontinue drug abruptly.
Captopril	Capoten	Available PO. Assess for tachycardia. May cause impotence. Administer 1 hour ac. Do not discontinue abruptly. May cause dizziness.
Clonidine	Catapres	Available PO/transdermal. Assess for hypotension, edema in extremities. Administer 1 hour ac. Photosensitivity is possible. Instruct patient about orthostatic hypotension.

Generic	Trade	Comments
Enalapril maleate	Vasotec	Available PO. Numerous GI side effects. Assess for hypotension. Instruct patient concerning orthostatic hypotension.
Guanethidine monosulfate	Ismelin	Available PO. Assess for hypotension, urinary retention. Instruct patient concerning orthostatic hypotension. Do not discontinue drug abruptly. Therapeutic response achieved in 1-2 weeks.
Hydralazine	Apresoline Dralzine	May be given PO, IM, IV. Take same way each time (i.e., with or without food). When giving IM, check BP every 5 minutes until stable. Headache and palpitations may occur with first dose.
Metoprolol	Lopressor Betaloc	May be given PO. Recommended to be taken with food. Take apical pulse before administering, hold if less than 60. Maximum effect seen in 1 week. Avoid exposure to cold. Medication should not be withdrawn.

Generic	Trade	Comments
Nitroprus-side sodium	Nipride Nitropress	Available IV. Rapid onset. Use infusion pump only. Monitor therapeutic effect closely. Incompatible with many drugs, do not mix with other drugs.
Propranolol	Inderal Novopranol	May be given PO, IV. Recommended before meals and bedtime. Tablet may be crushed. Take apical pulse before administering; hold drug, call physician if below 60. Monitor ECG, if given by

ANTI-INFECTIVES: AMINOGLYCOSIDES

ACTION: Bacterial action achieved by binding to the 30S ribosomal subunit, thereby inhibiting protein synthesis.

USES: Generally severe infections caused by sensitive *Pseudomonas aeruginosa, E. coli, Proteus, Klebsiella, Serratia, Enterobacter, Actinobacter, Staphylococcus,* consult your drug reference for specifics.

GENERAL COMMENTS: Always ascertain allergies prior to administration of first dose. Obtain culture and sensitivity prior to administration of first dose. Otoxicity has been associated with aminoglycocides to include vertigo, tinnitus, and hearing loss. Additionally, IV loop diuritics can increase the degree of ototoxicity. As with other anti-infectives watch for superinfection. Nephrotoxicity of varying degrees can occur. Ototoxicity may be obscured by concurrent use of dimenphydrinate. Therapy with cephalothin increases nephrotoxicity, also use caution when using with other aminoglycosides, amphotericin B, cisplatin, or methoxyflurane intensifies nephrotoxicity. Parenteral penicillins will inactivate aminoglycosides if mixed together.

Examples of Drugs in This Classification:

Generic	Trade	Comments
Amikacin sulfate	Amikin	Available IV or IM. Headache and lethargy may occur--use with caution in neonates, children, elderly or debilitated due to nephrotoxicity. Obtain weight and baseline renal function prior to initial therapy. Observe closely for signs and symptoms of decreasing renal function. Observe for signs or symptoms of ototoxicity such as decreased hearing, tinnitus or vertigo. Draw peak 1 hour after IM injection and 30 minutes to 1 hour after IV infusion. Draw trough level just prior to next dose.
Gentamycin sulfate	Garamycin Jenamicin	Available IV or IM. Headache and lethargy have occurred-use caution with therapy in neonates, children, elderly or debilitated due to nephrotoxicity. Obtain weight and baseline renal

Generic	Trade	Comments
		function prior to initiating therapy-monitor renal functions during therapy. Observe for signs or symptoms of ototoxicity such as decreased hearing, tinnitus or draw gentamycin peak 1 hour after IV infusion. Draw trough level just prior to next dose.
Neomycin sulfate	Mycifradin sulfate	Available PO, not recommended for IM use due to increased danger of ototoxicity and nephrotoxicity. Used PO to suppress intestinal bacteria prior to abdominal surgery. Headache and lethargy can occur. Watch for ototoxicity and nephrotoxicity. Obtain weight and baseline renal functions prior to initiating therapy. GI upset may occur.
Streptomycin sulfate	Same	Available IM. Watch for signs and symptoms of ototoxicity. Nephrotoxicity not as pronounced as other aminoglycosides. Exfolitative dermatitis has occurred. May be used for endocarditis, tuleremia.

Generic	Trade	Comments
		Primary and alternate therapy for tuberculosis.
Tobramycin sulfate	Nebcin	Available IM or IV. Headache and lethargy have been reported. Watch for signs and symptoms of ototoxicity and nephrotoxicity. Obtain weight and baseline renal functions prior to initiating therapy. Obtain peak levels one hour after IM injection and 30 minutes to 1 hour after IV infusion. Draw trough level prior to next dose.

ANTI-INFECTIVES: ANTIFUNGALS

ACTION: Binds to sterols in fungal cell membranes, therapy alters cell permeability facilitating intracellular leakage. Griseofulvins disrupt mitotic spindle structure.

USES: Systemic fungal infections such as histoplasmosis, coccidiomycosis, and others are treated with amphotericin. Topical fungi such as ringworm infections of skin, hair, nails are treated with griseofulvin. Additionally nystatin oral is used to treat vaginal and intestinal infections caused by *Candida*.

GENERAL COMMENTS: Specimen obtained for C & S prior to first dose if possible, identification of organism involved should be verified prior to continuing treatment. Antifungals vary in their applications, therefore a drug handbook should be consulted for specific information.

Examples of Drugs in This Classification:

Generic	Trade	Comments
Am-photericin B	Fungizone	Available IV. Permanent renal impairment may result from large doses. Monitor I & 0 closely. Administer IV preparation in distal veins to facilitate site rotation. Reconstitute only with sterile water to avoid precipitation.
Microsize Griseofulvin Ultramicrosize	FulvicinU/F Grifulvin U Guluicin P/G Grisactin Ultra Gris-PEG	Available PO. Varying CNS effects. Effects range from headache and fatigue to transient hearing loss and confusion; leukopenia may occur, draw regular CBC and discontinue if needed. Most effectively absorbed and causes the least GI distress when given with high-fat meals. Penicillin derivitive, use cautiously in patients sensitive to penicillin.
Nystatin	Mycostatin Milstat O-V Statin	Available PO. Virtually nontoxic and nonsensitizing. Not used for systemic infections.

ANTI-INFECTIVES: CEPHALOSPORINS

ACTION: Bactericidal and facilitates osmotic instability by inhibiting cell wall synthesis.

USES: Infections of urinary tract, blood, bone, joint, CNS, respiratory tract, skin, soft tissue, intraabdominal and gynecological infections caused by *Streptococci, E. coli, Proteus, Klebsiella, Staphylococci, N. gonorrhoea, Hemophilus influenzae, Enterobacter.*

GENERAL COMMENTS: Always ascertain allergies prior to administration of first dose. Caution advised when administering to patients with known sensitivity to penicillin and patients with impaired renal function. Observe for superinfection, because prolonged therapy can lead to overgrowth of nonsusceptible organisms, usually genital monilia and oral candida. Obtain culture and sensitivity prior to administration of first dose. Therapy may be initiated while culture and sensitivity is in progress. Probenecid may increase blood levels of cephalosporins by inhibiting their excretion. IM: inject deep into large muscle mass. Provide frequent IV assessments to decrease possibility of phlebitis and tissue sloughing.

Examples of Drugs in This Classification:

Generic	Trade	Comments
Cefamandole Nafate	Mandol	Available IM or IV. Various blood dyscrasias can occur. Headache, malaise possible-various GI adverse reactions possible-phlebitis and thromboplebitis can occur. Consuming alcohol may result in disulfiram-like reaction. Chemically incompatible with magnesium or calcium. Clinitest may read false positive.

Generic	Trade	Comments
Cefazolin sodium	Ancef Kefzol	Available IM or IV. Sometimes used as a perioperative prophylaxis. Various blood dyscrasias possible. Headache, malaise may occur. Various GI disturbances can occur. Phlebitis and thrombophlebitis may occur at IV site. Avoid therapy with greater than four grams per day in patients who have severely compromised renal function. IV administration results are best achieved with small gauge needle in large viens. Clinitest may read false positive.
Cefotaxime sodium	Claforan	Available IM or IV. Various blood dyscrasias, headache/malaise paresthesias and dizziness are common. Various GI disturbances can occur. Tissue sloughing and thrombophlebitis as well as phlebitis at injection and IV sites have occurred. Drug has increased antibacterial action against gram-negative micro-organisms. Not effective against Pseudomonas.

Generic	Trade	Comments
		Clinitest may read false positive.
Cefoxitin sodium	Mefoxin	Available IM or IV. Various blood dyscrasias can occur. Headache, malaise, paresthesias and dizziness have been reported. Various GI disturbances are possible. Pain at injection site with tissue sloughing and sterile abcesses are possible. Assess IV site frequently. Thrombophlebitis and phlebitis from IV use have been reported. Especially effective against *B. fragilis.* May be reconstituted with plain 5% or 19% lidocaine if ordered to minimize pain and discomfort from injection. May produce false positive clinitest.
Ceftazidime	Fortaz Tazicef Tazidime	Available IM or IV. Various blood dyscrasias can occur. Headache and dizziness occasionally reported. Various GI disturbances may occur. Transient increase in liver enzymes have been observed. Frequent IV site assessments are

Generic	Trade	Comments
		encouraged. Has longest half-life of any cephalosporin, may administer once per day. Renal toxicity not as pronounced as other cephalosporins. Used commonly in home antibiotic regimens such as osteomyelitis.
Cephalexin Monohydrate	Keflex	Available PO. Various transient blood dyscrasias have been reported. Dizziness, headache, malaise and paresthesias can occur. GI disturbances are possible. Instruct patient to complete all medication as prescribed even if symptoms have subsided. May take with food or milk to decrease GI disturbances. Clinitest may indicate false positive.
Cephalothin sodium	Keflin Seffin	Available IM or IV. Transient blood dyscrasias possible. Headache, malaise, dizziness and paresthesias have been reported. Various GI disturbances can occur. Medication is nephrotoxic. Frequent IV site assessments advised. Avoid

Generic	Trade	Comments
		IM route if possible. False positive clinitest can occur.
Cephradine	Anspor Uelosef	Available PO, IM, or IV. Transient minor blood dyscrasias possible. Headache, malaise, dizziness and paresthesias have been reported. Numerous GI disturbances can occur. Frequent IV site assessment advised. If prescribed PO, instruct patient to complete all medication as ordered even if symptoms subside. Follow reconstitution instructions precisely. This preparation is the only cephalosporin available in oral and injectable forms. Clinitest may read false positive.

ANTI-INFECTIVES: PENICILLINS

ACTION: Inhibits cell wall synthesis during active replication.

USES: Lower and upper respiratory tract infections, otitis media, sinusitis, UTI, and systemic infections caused by susceptible strains of gram-positive and gram-negative organisms. Systemic infections caused by penicillinase-producing Staphylococci, syphilis. Consult your drug reference for specifics.

GENERAL COMMENTS: Always ascertain allergies as cross-sensitivity is possible, especially cephalosporins. Rash is a common allergic reaction. Obtain specimen for C&S prior to first dose if possible. Give penicillins one hour before bacteriostatic antibiotics. Super-infections are possible. Penicillins are numerous and vary in their applications, therefore a drug handbook should be employed for specific information. Finish all PO medication as prescribed. Probenecid acts to increase serum levels of Penicillin. Always check expiration dates.

Examples of Drugs in This Classification:

Generic	Trade	Comments
Amoxicillin Trihydrate	Amoxil Larotid Polymox Trimox Robamox Ultimox Wymox	Available PO. Use cautiously when cross-sensitivity is a possibility. Teach patient to take all medication as prescribed. Take with food to prevent GI distress. Clinitest tablets may indicate false positive. Clinistix and Tes-Tape are not affected. Penicillins should be administered one hour prior to giving bacteriostatic antibiotics.
Ampicillin	Amcap Amcill D-Amp Pfizerpen Principen	Some available PO, IM, IV. Blood dyscrasias may occur. Nausea, vomiting and diarrhea are possible. Allergic reactions and cross-sensitivity are possible.

Generic	Trade	Comments
		Give one or two hours before meals or two to three hours after meals. Give IM or IV if ordered, only if patient cannot tolerate PO. Can cause false positive with clinitest tablets. Clinistix and Tes-Tape are not affected.
Ampicillin sodium	Omnipen Pen A/N	
Dicloxacillin sodium	Dycill Dynapen Pathocil	Available PO. Eosinophilia is possible. GI disturbance occasionally occurs. Allergic reactions and cross-sensitivity is possible. Rash is a common allergy.
Methicillin sodium	Staphcillin	Available IM or IV. Transient blood dyscrasias may occur. Neuropathy or siezures may occur with high doses. Glossitis or stomititis may occur. Intestitial nephritis is possible. Thrombophlebitis or vein irritation may occur. Allergic reaction and cross-sensitivity are possible. If ordered, give every 6 hours including night doses. Monitor renal function frequently.

Generic	Trade	Comments
		Reconstitute with a normal saline solution only. Change IV site every 48 hours.
Nafcillin sodium	Nafcil Nallpen Unipen	Available PO, IM, IV. Transient blood dyscrasias are possible. GI distress may occur. Thrombophlebitis or vein irritation is possible with IV administration. Allergic reaction and cross-sensitivity are possible. Mix only with dextrose 5% in water or a saline solution for KVO. Change IV site every 48 hours.
Penicillin G-Benzathine	Bicillin L-A Megacillin Suspension Permapen	Available IM. Transient dyscrasias are possible. Neuropathy and seizures are possible with high doses. Shake medication well before injection. Never give IV: Accidental IV administration has precepitated cardiac arrest and death. Give deep IM: Upper outer quadrant in adults only and in the midlateral thigh in infants and small children.

Generic	Trade	Comments
Penicillin G Potassium	Burcillin-G Delta pen Pentids	Available PO, IM, or IV. Transient blood dyscrasias are possible. Neuropathy and seizures are possible with high doses. Severe hyperkalemin possible with high doses. Thrombophlebitis and irritation at injection site is possible. May cause GI disturbance. Give one to two hours before meals or two to three hours after meals. Painful when administered IM. Give deep IM in large muscle. Change IV site every 48 hours. Administer IV only with dextrose 5% in water or a saline solution.
Penicillin G Procaine	Crysticillin-A.S. Duracillin-A.S. Pfizerpen-A.S.Wycillin	Available IM only. Transient blood dyscrasias are possible. Do not administer to patients allergic to procaine. Give deep IM only. Never give IV--Accidental administration has caused death related to CNS toxicity from procaine.
Penicillin V Penicillin V-Potassium	Betapen-V K Deltapen V K V-Cillin K	Available PO. Transient blood dyscrasias are possible. GI distress is possible. Sometimes given

Generic	Trade	Comments
		as endocarditis prophylaxis for dental surgery. Take with water. Fruit juice or carbonated beverage may inactivate drug due to acidity. Available IM or IV. Hemorrhage can occur with high dosage. Other transient blood dyscrasias are possible. Headache, neuromuscular irritability, dizziness are possible. GI disturbance is possible. Pain at injection site and thrombophlebitis possible. Hypokalemia has occurred. Chemically incompatible with aminoglycosides. Change IV site every 48 hours.
Piperacillin	Pipracil	Available IM or IV. Hemorrhage can occur with high dose. Other transient blood dyscrasias are possible. Headache, neuromuscular irritability, dizziness are possible. GI disturbance is possible. Pain at injection site and thrombophlebitis possible. Hypokalemia has occurred. Chemically incompatible with aminoglycosides.

Generic	Trade	Comments
Ticarcillin disodium	Ticar	Available IM or IV. Transient blood dyscrasias may occur. Seizures or neuromuscular irritability are possible with high doses. GI disturbances may occur. Hypokalemia is possible. Thrombophlebitis and pain at injection site may occur. Chemically incompatible with aminoglycosides. Usually used in combination with another antibiotic. Change IV site every 48 hours.

ANTI-INFECTIVES: TETRACYCLINES

ACTIONS: Binds to the 30S ribosomal subunit of affected microorganisms, inhibiting protein synthesis.

USES: Infections related to sensitive gram-negative and gram-positive bacteria as well as Trachoma, Rickettsia, Mycoplasma, Chlamydia and Amebiasis.

GENERAL COMMENTS: Always ascertain allergies prior to administration of first dose. Observe for superinfection, prolonged therapy may lead to overgrowth of non-susceptible organisms usually oral monilia. Obtain culture and sensitivity prior to administration of first dose of medication. Photosensitivity may occur with therapy. Antacids and laxatives containing aluminum, calcium or magnesium, inhibit absorption of these drugs, give dose 1 hour before or 2 hours after these drugs. Ferrous sulfate, zinc and other iron products decrease absorption, give dose

2 hours before or 3 hours after these drugs. Therapy during last half of pregnancy, as well as in children younger than 8 years old may cause discoloration of teeth, enamel defects or retardation of bone growth, do not use.

Examples of Drugs in This Classification:

Generic	Trade	Comments
Doxycycline hyclate	Doxy-Caps Doxy-Tabs Vibramycin Vibra Tabs Vivox	Available PO or IV. Sometimes prescribed as prophylaxis for "travelers diarrhea". Vibra Tabs: May cause transient blood dyscrasias. Various GI disturbances may occur. May take with food or milk if GI upset occurs. May be used in patients with renal impairment. Injectable may cause false positive clinitest. All forms can lead to false negative clinitest and test-tape. To prevent dysphagia, give more than one hour before bedtime.
Tetracycline hydrochloride	Achromycin	Available PO, IM, or IV. May cause various transient blood dyscrasias. Various GI distrubances have occurred. Can become hepatotoxic if given in large doses. BUN may increase. Thromboplebitis at IV site or irritation at injection site may occur. Do not

Generic	Trade	Comments
		mix with any other IV additive. When administering IM, inject deep in large muscle mass-tell patient drug be painful. This drug may be used via chest tube as a pleura sclerosing agent in malignant pleural effusions. Can cause false negative clinitest and test-tape.

ANTINEOPLASTICS: ALKYLATING AGENTS

ACTION: Effects cellular DNA by cross-linking strands resulting in cellular growth imbalance leading to cellular demise.

USES: Effective against metastatic carcinoma of the pancreas, colon cancer, cancers of breast, lung and ovaries, diffuse lymphocytic lymphoma, Hogdkin's disease, myelocytic leukemia, melanomas and various other neoplastic conditions. Uses vary, consult drug handbook for specifics.

GENERAL COMMENTS: Generally these agents have side effects which can include: nausea, vomiting, malaise, blurred vision, renal tubular necrosis, tissue damage at IV sites, peripheral neuropathy, alopecia, stomatitis, diarrhea, anorexia, peripheral edema and some mental changes. Laboratory tests may indicate thrombocytopenia, leukopenia or liver changes.   Always ascertain possible allergic conditions prior to administration.

Examples of Drugs in This Classification:

Generic	Trade	Comments
Cisplatin	Cis-Platinum II Platinol	Available IV. Used for testicular, ovarian and bladder cancer. Laboratory may show elevated BUN and creatinine. Monitor IV site for signs and symptoms of Monitor closely for hypothermia. May cause ototoxicity, monitor for changes in auditory function.
Cytoxin	Cyclophos-phamide	Available PO or IV. Monitor for evidence of bone marrow suppression. Used for lymphoma, multiple myecoma, leukemia, neuroblastoma, adenocarcinoma of the ovary. Can cause hemorrhagic cystitis. monitor for hematuria or dysuria. Monitor IV site for signs and symptoms of infiltration. Administer PO dose on empty stomach.
Dacarbazine	Dtic-Dome	Available IV. Used for malignant melanoma, Hodgkin's disease, sarcomas, neuroblastoma. Monitor I & O closely. Antiemetic is generally given for vomiting.

Generic	Trade	Comments
		Monitor IV site for signs and symptoms of infiltration.

ANTINEOPLASTICS: ANTIMETABOLITES

ACTION: These agents act by inhibiting pyrimidine synthesis or in the case of methotrexate, agent binds to dihydrofolate reductase preventing the reduction of folic acid to tetrahydrofolate.

USES: Effective against trophoblastic tumors, colon, rectal, breast, ovarian, bladder, cervical, pancreatic and liver cancers.   Additionally, used against myelocytic leukemia. Uses vary with agents, consult your drug handbook for specifics.

GENERAL COMMENTS: These agents have side effects which can include: nausea, vomiting, anorexia, alopecia, potential for hemorrhage, malaise, jaundice, edema of lower extremities, possible severe CNS complications. May lead to leukopenia and thrombocytopenia.   Also these agents can cause photosensitivity.   Always ascertain possible allergic conditions prior to administration.

Examples of Drugs in This Classification.

Generic	Trade	Comments
Cytarabine	Cytosar-V	Available IV. Used for malignant leukemia. Monitor for signs and symptoms of adverse and side effects. Nephrotoxic, insure adequate hydration. Monitor I&O. Frequent CNS assessments. Monitor

Generic	Trade	Comments
		IV site for signs and symptoms of infiltration.
Fluorouracil	Adrucil F-FU 5-Fluorouracil	Available PO, topical, IV. Used for cancer of breast, colon, liver, stomach, ovary, basal cell cancer. Monitor laboratory results for blood dyscrasias. Assess frequently for adverse reactions. Monitor IV site for signs and symptoms of infiltration.
Methotrexate sodium	Folex Mexate	Available PO, IM, IV. Used for trophoblastic tumors, lymphatic leukemia, meningeal leukemia, stage III, lymphosarcoma stage I or stage II Burkitt's lymphoma. May be extremely neurotoxic. Frequent CNS assessments. Monitor for hemorrhage. Increase fluid intake as ordered to promote adequate hydration. May cause photosensitivity. Monitor IV site for signs and symptoms of infiltration.

ANTINEOPLASTICS: ANTIBIOTIC AGENTS

ACTION: These agents interfere with DNA synthesis in a variety of ways, by strand splitting; by interference with RNA synthesis and ultimately protein synthesis.

USES: Effective against cancers of the cervix, esophagus, head, neck and testes. Also used in Hodgkin's disease, lymphomas, sarcomas, leukemia, neuroblastoma and Wilm's tumor. Applications of agents in this classification may be drug specific, dosages and and indications vary, consult your drug handbook for specifics.

GENERAL COMMENTS: These agents have many potential adverse reactions, including multiple dermatalogical problems ranging from rash to desquamation of hands and feet, increased tactile sensitivity especially to pressure and pain, nausea, stomatitis, reversible alopecia, leukopenia, thrombocytopenia, anorexia and locally severe tissue damage from extravasation. Some agents may be hepatotoxic. A variety of CNS problems have occasionally occurred, including anxiety, depression, confusion and rarely hallucinations. Always access for allergic conditions prior to administration.

Examples of Drugs in This Classification:

Generic	Trade	Comments
Bleomycin	Blenoxane	Available SC, IM, IV. Causes various blood dyscrasias. May cause various pulmonary complications. Use cautiously in pulmonary impaired patients. Onset of allergic reactions may take up to 5 hours past

Generic	Trade	Comments
		administration. This drug may post administration. Monitor IV site frequently.
Daunorubicin hydrochloride	Cerubidine	Available IV. Blood dyscrasias may occur. May be nephrotoxic. Will cause benign transient red urine, explain to patient. Frequent IV assessment.
Doxorubicin	Adriamycin ADR	Available IV. Effective against Wilm's tumor. May cause severe blood dyscrasias. Will cause benign transient red urine, explain to patient.

ANTINEOPLASTICS: MISCELLANEOUS AGENTS

ACTION: These agents achieve therapeutic results in a wide variety of ways, mostly drug specific.

USES: Effective against acute lymphocytic leukemia, Hodgkin's disease, lymphosarcoma, neuroblastoma, Wilm's tumor and breast cancer.   Applications vary greatly. Consult your drug handbook for specifics.

GENERAL COMMENTS: These agents have many adverse reactions associated with their administration, be throughly familiar with specific agents being utilized. Mostly administered in hospital settings.

Examples of Drugs in This Classification:

Generic	Trade	Comments
Asparaginase	Elspar	Available IM, IV. May cause Hypofibrinoginase-enemia and depression of other monitor coagulation functions. Usually used in conjunction with additional agents. May cause severe nausea and vomiting. Monitor IV sites frequently.
Vincristine sulfate	Oncovin	Available IV. Causes mild blood dyscrasias. Multiple CNS adverse reactions reported, do frequent neuroassessments. May cause constipation. Acute, life threatening bronchospasm has occurred. Monitor IV site frequently.

ANTI-INFLAMMATORIES

ACTION: Decreases or prevents inflammation of joints.

USES: Arthritis, including juvenile, adult, rheumatoid, or other disorders where inflammation of the joints is a problem.

GENERAL COMMENTS: Drugs shown here vary widely, and a drug handbook should be consulted prior to administering gold compounds. Over-the-counter drug use with these medications should be checked with physician.

Examples of Drugs in This Classification:

Generic	Trade	Comments
Aurothio-glucose	Solganal	May be given deep IM. Used to treat rheumatoid arthritis. Many adverse side effects. Stomatitis may occur.
Gold sodium thiomalate	Myochrysine	May be given IM. Used to treat rheumatoid arthritis.
Ibuprofen	Motrin Advil Nuprin	May be given PO. Used to treat rheumatoid arthritis, osteoarthritis, musculo-skeletal pain. Take on empty stomach for best results. Tablet may be crushed and mixed with food or drink. Available over-the-counter.
Oxyphen-butazone	Oxalid	May be given PO. Tablet may be crushed and mixed with food. Administer with food.

ANTILIPEMICS

ACTION: To lower blood cholesterol, fat levels.

USES: High serum cholesterol and fat levels that have not responded to dietary interventions.

GENERAL COMMENTS: High cholesterol and fat levels have been associated with cardiovascular disease.

Examples of Drugs in This Classification:

Generic	Trade	Comments
Choles-tyramine	Questran	Available PO. Many drug interactions. Assess bowel pattern daily. Observe for hemorrhage. Compliance to regimen necessary since toxicity may result if doses are missed. Avoid OTC preparations.
Clofibrate		Available PO. Multiple GI disturbances may occur. Assess bowel pattern daily. Compliance to regimen necessary since toxicity may result if doses are missed.
Lovastatin	Mevacor	Dosage is adjusted at 4 week intervals depending on patient response. Low incidence of side effects.

ANTIPSYCHOTICS

ACTION: Postsynaptic dopamine receptors in brain are blocked.

USES: Predominantly used for psychosis.

GENERAL COMMENTS: A high incidence of CNS adverse reactions occur including: EPS, sedation, dizziness and tardive dyskinesia. Anticholinergic side effects that are common are constipation, dry mouth, urinary retention. Various drug interactions require caution, antacids inhibit absorption of PO phenothiazines, give a least 2 hours apart. Anticholinergic drugs compound   these   effects   in antipsychotics.   Barbituates may decrease phenothiazine effect.   Do not combine with alcohol.   Orthostatic hypotension is common. Generally contraindicated in coma, subcortical damage, CNS depression. Use with caution in elderly or debilitated patients and in children.   Tardive dyskinesia is associated with long term use, onset may be rapid or not appear for years and is not reversible. Phenothiazines are associated with photosensitivity. Weight gain may occur.

Examples of Drugs in this Classification:

General	Trade	Comments
Chlorproma-zine HCl	Chlorizine Ormazine Promaz Thorazine	Available PO, IM, suppositories. Aliphatic phenothiazine. May be used for intractable hiccups, or alcohol withdrawal as well as psychosis. Possible decreased therapeutic action when administered with lithium. May lower seizure threshold. Various blood dyscrasias can occur. Assess for urinary retention. Advise patients to use sunscreen when outdoors. Frequent assessment of V/S. Give deep IM.
Fluphenazine Decanoate/ Fluphenazine HCl Fluphenazine Enanthate	Prolixin Decanoate Prolixin HCl Prolixin Enanthate	Available IM, SC. A piperazine phenothiazine. Monitor CBC and hepatic functions. Requires 24-96 hours for initial therapeutic response.

General	Trade	Comments
		In decanoate and enanthate administer q-3wks.
Haloperidol Haloperidol Decanoate	Haldol Haldol Decanoate	Available PO, IM. Adverse drug interactions with lithium, and methyldopa. Common therapy for agitation in senile dementia. Caution not to administer decanoate IV.
Loxapine	Loxitane Loxitane-C	Available PO or IM. A dibenzoxazepine. Transient blood dyscrasias possible. No significant drug interactions. Liquid may be diluted with fruit juice.
Molindone HCl	Moban	Available PO. A dihydroindolone. Transient blood dyscrasias possible. Assess for urinary retention. No significant drug interactions. May be given as a single daily dose.
Perphenazine	Trilafon	Available PO or IM. Monitor CBC and hepatic functions. Give deep IM. Assess for urinary retention. Dilute liquid concentrate with fruit juices.
Thioridazine HCl	Mellaril Millazine	Available PO. A piperidine phenothiazine. Transient blood dyscrasias occur.

Generic	Trade	Comments
		Monitor CBC and hepatic functions. Assess for urinary retention. May dilute liquid concentrate in fruit juice.
Thiothixene	Navane	A thioxanthene. Available PO or IM. Can lead to blood dyscrasias. Monitor CBC and hepatic function. Assess for urinary retention. Assess for orthostatic hypotension. Give deep IM. May mix oral liquid concentrate with fruit juice.
Triluo-perazine HCl Stelazine	Suprazine	Available PO or IM. Piperidine phenothiazine. Various blood dyscrasias possible. Assess for urinary retention. Monitor CBC and hepatic functions. May dilute PO liquid concentrate in fruit juice. Assess for orthostatic hypotension.

ANTITUSSIVES

ACTION: To suppress coughing, may be either narcotic or nonnarcotic.

USES: Non-productive cough or to provide relief for an overactive cough.

GENERAL COMMENTS: Narcotic anitussives are addictive, may cause constipation and drowsiness. Alcohol should be avoided while while taking this medication.

Examples of Drugs in This Classification:

Generic	Trade	Comments
Codeine	Codeine	May be given PO, SC, IM. Narcotic antiussive. Administer with food or milk to decrease GI distress. Nausea is a common side effect. Addiction and dependence may occur.
Dextro-methorphan hydrobomide	Hold Sucrets Creamcoat Mediquell Robitussin DM	Non-narcotic antitussive. May be given PO. May be purchased over-the-counter.

ANTIULCER AGENTS

ACTION: Reduces gastric acid.

USES: Conditions where gastric acid needs to be reduced such as in gastric ulcers, duodenal ulcers, stress ulcers.

GENERAL COMMENTS: Antacids are often used concurrently with histamine blockers to treat ulcers.

Examples of Drugs in This Classification:

Generic	Trade	Comments
Cimetidine	Tagamet	May be taken PO, IV push, IV, IM. Administer with or just after meals. Administer antacids at least one hour before or after this drug. Many drug interactions.

Generic	Trade	Comments
Ranitidine	Zantac	May be taken PO. Long
Famotidine	Pepcid	term use may lead to B_{12}
Misoprostol	Cytotec	deficiency.
Nizatidine	Axid	
Omeprazole	Losec	

BRONCHODILATORS

ACTION: Relaxes bronchial muscle, reduces bronchial edema and mucous production.

USES: To control wheezing and improve activity tolerance by reducing respiratory symptoms. May be used in any of the following conditions: allergies, asthma, bronchitis, emphysema, hay fever, or any obstructive airway disease.

GENERAL COMMENTS: Bronchodilators increase cardiac rate and output. Palpitation, nervousness, restlessness, anxiety and hypertension are all possible side effects. Vital signs should be taken prior to and frequently during administaration by the parenteral routes. Bronchodilators given by the inhalation route are often misused, and patient should be instructed in the correct procedure, correct dosage and frequency of use.

Examples of Drugs in This Classification:

Generic	Trade	Comments
Ephedrine	Efedrin Vatronol	May be given SC, IM, IV slow, intranasal and topical. Common ingredient in over-the-counter cold/allergy medications. Check for drug interactions when multiple medications are ordered.

Generic	Trade	Comments
Epinephrine HCl	Adrenaline Sus-phrine Bronkaid Mist Primatene Mist	Always aspirate prior to injecting to prevent accidental IV administration of SC dose. Avoid buttocks for IM route. Cardiac monitor is recommended for IV use. One of the first line drugs in cardiac arrest. May be given by SC, inhalation, topical routes, IM, IV. Always check for correct route on orders and medication vial.
Isoproterenol HCl	Isuprel Norisodrine Proternol	May be given inhalation, SL, rectal, SC, IV, IC. Sublingual tablet may be given by rectal route if ordered. May be given via oxygen aerosal treatment. Do not administer with epinephrine, give at least 4 hours apart. May be given for cardiac arrest.
Metapro-terenol SO_4	Alupent Metaprel	Available PO, inhaler, aerosol. Effective against acute episodes of bronchial asthma. May cause anxiety, tachycardia. Paradoxical bronchiolar constriction may occur with excessive use.

Generic	Trade	Comments
Terbutaline SO$_4$	Brethine Brethaire Bricanyl	May be given by PO, SC, inhalation, IV routes. Tablets may be crushed. Tablets can be taken with food for GI upset.
Theophylline	Slo-bid Theo-Dur Bronkodyl Lano-phyllin	May be given PO. Therapeutic range is 10-20 mcg/ml. Enteric coated tablets should not be crushed (or sustained release tablets). Administer after meals with water to prevent GI irritation. Dizziness occurs frequently in early treatment.

CARDIAC GLYCOSIDES/INOTROPIC AGENTS

ACTION: Increases the force of cardiac contraction while slowing the heart rate.

USES: Congestive heart failure, cardiac arrhythmias, cardiogenic shock from cardiac trauma (myocardial infarction).

GENERAL COMMENTS: Take apical pulse prior to administration, hold drug if irregular or under 60 beats per minute. When potassium levels are low, there is increased sensitivity to this drug; potassium should be monitored in any patients. Cardiac glycosides are powerful drugs and should be stored away from small children, accidential ingestion may be lethal. A medical alert bracelet should be worn when taking these drugs.   Over-the-counter medications should not be taken without consulting physician.

Examples of Drugs in This Classification:

Generic	Trade	Comments
Amrinone Lactate	Inocor	Available IV. Inotropic action. Monitor for arrhythmias. Can be hepatotoxic. Precipitates with furosemide. Administer with infusion pump only.
Digoxin	Lanoxicaps Lanoxin	Not the same drug as digitoxin. May be given PO, IM, IV. Tablet may be crushed. Serum levels are required, therapeutic range is 0.8-2 mg/ml. IM route is associated with intense pain. Anorexia is a sign of toxicity. Weight daily, assess for edema. Store in light-resistant container.

CORTICOSTERIODS

ACTION: Act by stabilizing leukocytes lysosomal membranes, decreasing inflammation. Protein, fat, and carbohydrate metabolism is affected, immune response is suppressed and bone marrow is stimulated.

USES: Corticosteroids are used to combat severe inflammation, prevention of neonatal respiratory distress syndrome, adrenal insufficiency, allergic reactions, steroid-dependent asthma, systemic shock, as well as immunosuppression.

GENERAL COMMENTS: Generally contraindicated in systemic fungal infections, use caution in patients with GI ulceration, renal impairment, hypertension, osteoporosis, varicella, diabetes mellitus, Cushing's syndrome, CHF, metastatic carcinoma, tuberculosis, thromboembolic conditions, or herpes simplex. These drugs may mask infection leading to serious systemic infections. Potassium supplement may be necessary. Never discontinue drug abruptly. Teach patient signs and symptoms of adrenal insufficiency, including general malaise, joint pain, fever, anorexia, syncope, nausea, dyspnea. High dose therapy can lead to depression or psychotic episodes. Generally, patients on long term therapy bruise easily, observe closely for petechiae, GI upset reported with PO use. Patients undergoing long therapy should be instructed concerning Cushing symptoms. Interaction with barbiturates, phenytoin or rifampin decrease corticosteroid GI distress and bleeding increased with concurrent use of indomethacin and ASA.

Examples of Drugs in This Classification:

Generic	Trade	Comments
Belometh-asone Dipropionate	Beclovent Vanceril	Available as inhalant. Can lead to oral fungal infections. Dryness of mouth occurs. Dosage increase may be necessary in times of stress. If on inhaled bronchodilator, use several minutes prior to this medication. Insure patient understands this drug is not effective against acute asthma attack. Assess frequently

Generic	Trade	Comments
		for fungal infections of oral mucosa. Oral fungal infections may be diminished by following inhalations with a glass of water. Instruct patient to keep inhaler sanitary.
Cortisone Acetate	Cortistan Cortone	Available PO or IM. May need low sodium diet with potassium supplement. Slow onset of action with IM doses. Has increased mineralcorticoid effect, be alert for sudden weight gain, or edema. Corticosteroids may lead to delayed wound healing. This is the primary drug of choice in adrenal insufficiency as a replacement. To decrease toxicity, administer once per day in the AM. Not to be used IV.
Dexamethasone	Decadron Dexone Hexadrol Savacort-D	Available PO, IM, IV. Monitor weight and serum electrolytes. Give dose once per day in AM for reduced toxicity. May lead to delayed wound healing. Administer PO with food if possible. Currently used also to aid in diagnosis of

Generic	Trade	Comments
		depression. Can be an effective antiemetic.
Fludrocor-tisone Acetate	Florinef Acetate	Available PO. No significant drug interactions. Can lead to cardiac atrophy. Monitor weight and observe for edema. Used with cortisone or hydrocortisone, as partial replacement.
Hydrocor-tisone Sodium Suc-cinate Hydrocor-tisone Retention Enema	Cortef Hydrocor-tone A-Hydrocort Solu-Cortef Cortenema Rectoid	Available PO, IM, IV. Enemas used in treatment of ulcerative colitis. Glucocorticoid as well as mineral corticoid action. Monitor growth patterns in infants and children with long-term therapy. Give deep IM to avoid tissue atrophy. Monitor serum electrolytes. Be alert to same similarities; do not confuse Solu-Cortef with Solu-Medrol.
Methylpred-nisolone	Depo-Medrol Duralone Medrol	Available IM and IV. Decreased mineral corticoid effect. Monitor weight and electrolytes. Give deep IM. Administer IV slowly, over 10 minutes, to prevent circulatory collapse.

Generic	Trade	Comments
Prednisone	Deltasone Meticorten Orasone	Available PO. Monitor serum electrolytes and weight. Administer once daily in AM if possible. Give PO dose with food. Available in oral solution.

DECONGESTANTS

ACTION: Relieves nasal congestion.

USES: Allergies, upper respiratory infections, otitis media.

GENERAL COMMENTS: May have stimulant effects. Do not administer at bedtime. Often found in over-the-counter medications, especially antihistamines. Avoid mixing OTC drugs as action may be increased.

Examples of Drugs in This Classification:

Generic	Trade	Comments
Ephedrine	Efedron Vatronol	See bronchodilators. May produce sneezing, burning of nasal passages.
Oxymeta-zoline	Afrin Duration Neo-Synephrine Sinex	Available over-the-counter. Prolonged decongestant effect. Rebound congestion can occur with misuse. May be given by nasal drops.
Pseudo-ephedrine	Sudafed Sudabid	May be given by PO route. Tablets may be crushed. See also Ephedrine.

EMETICS

ACTION: Induces vomiting.

USES: Ingestion of toxic substance or drug overdose.

GENERAL COMMENTS: Prior to administration in suspected or known poisoning, poison control center should be notified of ingested substance as vomiting may be contraindicated.

Example of Drugs in This Classification:

Generic	Trade	Comments
Syrup of Ipecac		May be taken PO. Available over-the-counter. Should be taken with water. Do not administer with activated charcoal. Observe for abuse.

EXPECTORANTS

ACTION: Decreases the viscosity of respiratory secretions.

USES: Non-productive cough.

GENERAL COMMENTS: Use and therapeutic value are controversial. Any persistent cough should be evaluated for cause, as it may indicate a more severe problem. Increased fluid intake and humidification of air is recommended to augment effects.

Examples of Drugs in This Classification:

Generic	Trade	Comments
Acetylcys-teine	Mucomyst Parrolex	Available PO, solution. May cause bronchospasm, use cautiously in asthmatics. Monitor effectiveness: Assess quality of cough. Is a mucocytic.

Generic	Trade	Comments
Guaifenesin	Anti-Tuss Robitussin	May be given by PO route. Common ingredient of cough medications.

ESTROGENS

ACTION: DNA, RNA and protein synthesis are increased in target tissues. A reduction in FSH and LH release from the pituitary is achieved.

USES: In women; menopausal symptoms, female hypogonadism, atrophic vaginitis and kraurosis vulvae, primary ovarian failure, or surgical removal of ovaries, postpartum breast engorgement and breast cancer and occasionally osteoporosis. In men; prostatic cancer, breast cancer.

GENERAL COMMENTS: In general estrogens can have a wide variety of adverse effects including: Headache, migraine, depression, changes in libido, thromboembolism, increased risk of stroke, pulmonary embolism and myocardial infarction, intolerance to contact lenses, various GI disturbances, various adverse menstrual conditions, and in males impotence, gynecomastia and testicular atrophy. Cholestatic jaundice is reported. Additionally, hypercalcemia, hyperglycemia and folic acid deficiency have been reported. Various dermatological adverse effects can occur, such as acne, loss of hair, hirsutism and melasma. Estrogen therapy is contraindicated in patients with thrombophlebitis or thromboembolic conditions, and any undiagnosed genital bleeding. Caution should be exercised in patients with asthma, depression, blood dyscrasias, gall-bladder disease, migraine, diabetes mellitus, CHF or renal conditions. Insure patient has access to product information. Instruct patient about signs and symptoms of

thrombophlebitis or thromoboembolis. No significant drug
interactions reported. Use of estrogens linked to increased
incidence of breast and endometrial carcinoma.

Examples of Drugs in This Classification:

Generic	Trade	Comments
Chloro-trianisene	Tace	Available PO. Inform male patients concerning gynecomastia and impotence with long term therapy. Monitor blood glucose.
Diethylstil-bestrol	DES	Available PO. May be used for postcoital contraception only 25 mg tablet if approved for this application. Discontinue immediately if patient becomes pregnant during therapy. If specimen obtained for pathology, inform lab about therapy. Long term therapy for prostatic carcinoma has been linked to increased mortality from cardiovascular conditions. Inform male patients that gynecomastia and impotence will subside after therapy is discontinued.

Generic	Trade	Comments
Estradiol	Estrace Estrace vaginal cream Estraderm Depogen Dura Estrin	Available PO, vaginal cream and transdermal patch. No significant drug interactions reported. Monitor electrolytes, glucose. Inform male patients that gynecomastia and impotence will subside after therapy is discontinued. If specimens obtained for pathology inform lab of therapy.
Estrogenic-substances conjugated	Estrocon Premarin	Available PO, IM, or IV. No significant drug interactions reported. IM or IV route desirable to rapidly control severe uterine bleeding. Inform male patients that gynecomastia and impotence will subside after therapy is discontinued. If specimens obtained for pathology, notify lab of therapy.

LAXATIVES

ACTION: Aids in the passage of stool.

USES: Constipation, hard infrequent stools.

GENERAL COMMENTS: Laxative abuse is common, laxatives in general should be taken with fluids. Encourage diet high in fiber, increased fluids, exercise, to promote normal bowel function without laxatives. Laxative abuse can lead to dependence as the GI tract may lose ability to expel stool without medication.

Examples of Drugs in This Classification:

Bulk forming agents generally work in 12-24 hrs. but may take up to 72 hrs.

Generic	Trade	Comments
Psyllium	Metamucil Mucillium Mucilose Reguloid V-Lax	May be taken PO. May be mixed with water, fruit juice, milk or any liquid. Follow with 8 oz. of water for best results. Some products are high in sodium.

Fecal softener-Stool softened in 1-3 days

Docusate Calcium	Surfak	May increase absorption of other drugs, leading to toxicity at lower doses.
Docusate sodium	Colace DioSul Regutol	Sodium product should be avoided in patients with kidney or heart problems.

Hyperosmolar laxatives

Lactulose	Cephulac Chronulac	Works in 24-48 hrs. May be given PO. Avoid giving with meals due to taste. Given to detoxify ammonia in hepatic disorders. Avoid exposure to light.
Magnesium Salts	Milk of Magnesia, Magnesium Citrate, Citroma	Works in 2-6 hours. Avoid use in renal patients. Shake well. Give before meals or at bedtime.

Generic	Trade	Comments
Lubricants		
Mineral oil	Agoral plain	Do not take with food or medication, take with fruit juice. May be given PO, rectal route. Usually administered in evening.
Stimulant Irritant		
Bisacodyl	Dulcolax Deficol Theralax	May be given PO. Do not crush or chew tablets. Do not take with milk or antacids. Works in 1 hr.
Cascara sagrada		May change color of urine. Usually taken in evening. Works in 6-12 hrs.
Castor oil	Alphamul Emulsoil Neoloid Purge	May be given with juice for taste. Should be taken on an empty stomach. Works in 3 hrs.
Phenol-phthalein	Ex Lax Feen-A-Mint Prulet	Effect may last 3-4 days. Usually taken in the evening. Works in 6-12 hrs. May change color of urine. Discontinue if rash develops.

MUSCLE RELAXANTS

ACTION: Decreases unwanted involuntary movements and decreases muscle tone, often used to relieve muscular pain.

USES: Muscle strains, sprains, low back pain, arthritis, bursitis, multiple sclerosis.

GENERAL COMMENTS: Decreased mental alertness may occur with use of these medications. Instruct patient to avoid any hazardous activities such as driving or operating equipment until effect of medication is known. Over-the-counter medications should not be taken without checking with physician first. Instruct patient not to stop drug without medical supervision. Alcohol use should be avoided when taking these medications.

Examples of Drugs used in This Classification:

Generic	Trade	Comments
Baclofen	Lioresal Lioresal DS	May be given PO. Not to be used with CNS depressant. May be taken with food.
Carisoprodol	Rela Soma	May be given PO. Not to be used with CNS depressant. May be taken with food.
Chlor-phenesin Carbamate	Maolate	May be given PO. Monitor CBC. Not to be used with CNS depressant. Watch for sore throat, bleeding; blood dyscraisis may occur. Skeletal muscle relaxant.
Chlorzoxa-zone	Paraflex Oxyren	Given PO. Orange or purple urine may occur. Not to be used with CNS depressant.
Cycloben-zaprine	Flexeril	May be given PO. Dry mouth may be present. Short-term use drug.
Dantrolene sodium	Dantrium Dartrium IV	May be given PO, IV. Give IV after assessing for

Generic	Trade	Comments
		blood return, very irritating to tissue. Assess ambulation, as may be affected by this drug. Monitor for jaundice during use.
Methocar-bamol	Forbaxin Robamol Robaxin	No CNS depressants should be used. IV slowly. Urine may turn green or black. With meals for GI upset. Orthostatic hypotension may occur with IV. WBC count needed.
Or-phenadrine citrate	Banflex Norflex Myolin	Very toxic at high doses. Give IV over 5 minutes. Watch for high temperature, flushing, blurred vision, dry mouth, toxicity.

OXYTOCICS

ACTION: Promotes uterine contractions, to stimulate the flow of breast milk in the postpartum mother.

USES: Initiates or stimulates labor in selected term pregnancies, used for control of postpartum, to promote the letdown reflex in breast-feeding mothers.

GENERAL COMMENTS: Cautious use is required, these preparations may lead to fetal or maternal fatalities if used incorrectly. Constant supervision of patient during use is recommended. Assess for previous uterine surgery, cephalopelvic disproportion and fetal distress prior to use.

Pulse and blood pressure should be monitored frequently (q 15 min.) during use, fetal heart rate should be monitored continuously. This medication should never be used without a volume control-pump. Check all calculations and orders with another nurse. Assess for hypercontractility of the uterus in antepartum women and discontinue IV, turn client to left side, administer oxygen and notify physician.

Examples of Drugs in This Classification:

Generic	Trade	Comment
Carboprost tromethamine	Prostin/M15	May be given IM. Used to induce abortion in the 13-20th week of gestation. Monitor for pyrexia.
Ergonovine maleate	Ergotrate maleate	May be given PO, IM, IV. Used to prevent postpartum hemorrhage. Check orders for route and admission time prior to delivery.
Oxytocin	Pitocin Syntocinon Utercon	May be given IV drip or nasal spray or drops. Only one route should be used at any one time. Widely used for induction of labor as it stimulates muscular contraction of the uterus. IV infusion of 1 ml/1000 ml D_5W or 0.9% NaCl over 1-2 milli U/min; may increase q15-30 min., not to exceed 20 milli U/min.

HYPNOTICS/SEDATIVES

ACTIONS: Hypnotics promote sleep; sedatives promote relaxation, provide a calming effect.

USES: Hypnotics may be used at any time when the promotion of sleep is the goal such as for insomnia, as an aid prior to surgical procedures. Sedatives may be used to treat anxiety, acute reactions to stressful situations (grief reactions) and agitation.

GENERAL COMMENTS: The potential for dependence is high, use of medications should be temporary and monitored closely. Tolerance to drugs may develop requiring higher doses to achieve the same effect. Instruct patients not to give medication to others. Medication should not be administered to relieve pain. Alcohol and other medications that depress the CNS should be avoided.

Examples of Drugs in This Classification:

Generic	Trade	Comments
Amobarbital	Amytal Isobec	May be given PO, IM, IV. Sedative and hypnotic. May be given in status epilepticus.
Chloral hydrate	Cohidrate Noctec	May be given PO, rectal. Often used as a sedative/hypnotic in children and elderly. Administer after meals to prevent GI upset.
Flurazepam	Dalmane Durapan	May be given PO. Capsules may be opened and contents mixed with food or fluids.

Generic	Trade	Comments
Paraldehyde	Paral	May be given PO, rectal, IM, IV. May be used in alcohol withdrawal for sedation. Reported to have unpleasant taste, administer in juice or milk to improve taste and help prevent GI upset. Discard unused portion of unit container after 24 hours. Do not use if vinegar odor is noted. Inject IM deep, in UOQ.
Phenobar- bital	Bar Eskabarb Floramine	May be given PO, rectal, IM, IV.
Secobarbital	Seconal	Hypnotic/sedative. May be given as a premedication prior to spinal or regional anesthesia.
Temazepam	Restoril	May be given PO. Used primarily for early morning awakening, not for difficulty in falling asleep. May aggravate confusion in elderly.
Triazolam	Halcion	May be given PO. Hypnotic. Usually no daytime effects are present. Used for short term man- agement of insomnia. Smoking decreases effective- ness of this medication.

PROGESTERONES

ACTION: It is believed that by inhibiting pituitary gonadtropin secretion that these drugs act to inhibit ovulation; additionally, a thick cervical mucus is formed.

USES: Various menstrual irregularities, uterine cancer, uterine bleeding related to hormonal imbalance, endometrial or renal carcinoma, amenorrhea, endometriosis, management of PMS.

GENERAL COMMENTS: Serious cardiovascular conditions have occurred with therapy including thrombophlebitis, hypertension, pulmonary embolism and severe edema. Headache and migraine as well as depression have been reported. Various GI upset can occur. Breast tenderness, discharge or enlargement may occur. Uterine fibromas, abnormal secretions and breakthrough bleeding have been reported. Cholestatic jaundice can occur, as can hyperglycemia and decreased libido. Contraindicated in vaginal bleeding which has not been diagnosed, thromboembolic disorders, pregnancy, hepatic conditions. Exercise caution when diabetes mellitus is present as well as cardiac and renal impairments. Use cautiously in patients with asthma or migraine conditions. Regulations of FDA mandate that prior to administration of first dose patients are instructed to read product information insert.

Examples of Drugs in This Classification:

Generic	Trade	Comments
Medroxypro-gesterone acetate	Amen Curretab Depo-Provera Provera	Available PO or IM. IM injection may be painful. Not to be used as a test for pregnancy, may cause

Generic	Trade	Comments
		birth defects. In obstructive sleep apnea, has been effective.
Norethin-drone acetate	Aygestin Norlutate	Available PO. Generally in menstrual disorders preliminary estrogen therapy may be needed. This drug is twice as potent as plain norethindrone.
Progesterone	Femotrone Profac-O Progelan Progest-50 Progestaject-50 Progestasert	Available IM, intrauterine device or suppository. Give deep IM. Assess for proper IUD placement. IUD dosage good for one year only. Inform patient of potential complications of intrauterine devices

VASODILATORS

ACTION: Relaxes smooth muscle, producing vasodilation which decreases amount of blood returned to the heart and thereby decreases cardiac output.

USES: Angina, also used with blood pressure medications.

GENERAL COMMENTS: Headaches are common the first few days of treatment, BP should be monitored prior to administration for postural hypotension. Medical alert bracelet should be worn.

Examples of Drugs in This Classification:

Generic	Trade	Comments
Cyclandelate	Cyclospasmol Cyclan	Available PO. Monitor bleeding time. Administer with meals. Dizziness may occur. Stress compliance.
Dipyridamole	Persantine Pyridamole	Used for chronic angina. May be taken PO. Take 1 hour before, or 2 hours after meals. Tablets may be crushed.
Isoxsuprine HCl	Vasodilan Voxsupine	Available PO. Monitor orthostatic blood pressures. May cause dizziness. Instruct patient about orthostatic hypotension.
Nylidrin HCl	Arlidin Rolidrin	Available PO. Monitor orthostatic blood pressures. Instruct patient about orthostatic hypotension. Stress compliance since therapeutic response may take 2-3 months. May cause dizziness.

VITAMINS

A vitamin is an organic compound derived from the diet and needed in very small quantities to promote growth and maintain life. The following tables have been included to provide information on each of 13 major vitamins. The first four vitamins are fat soluble and are insoluble in water. They are A, D, E, and K.

VITAMIN A

RDA	800-1,000 ug RE
Principle sources	Egg yolk, liver, lamb chops, milk, butter. Yellow-orange pigment foods: Apricots, cantaloupe, peaches, carrots, sweet potatoes, yellow squash. Green vegetables: Broccoli, spinach
Function in body	Night vision, mucous secretions, formation of cartilage, growth and repair of cells, needed for spermatogenesis.
Storage in body	Liver
Overdose symptoms	Greater than 100,000 ug RE/day for 2-3 weeks; lethargy, abdominal pain, headache, sweating, joint pain, jaundice and loss of hair.
Deficiency symptoms	Night blindness, spots, xerophthalmia, blindness, UTI, diarrhea.
Persons at risk	Elderly, infants, diabetics, alcoholics, smokers, drug addicts, and persons with hyperthyroidism.
Antagonists	Air pollution, strong light, mineral oil, or increased protein intake

Synergists	Vitamins D, E, and C
Comments	Carotene is the precursor to Vitamin A, fat soluble and insoluble in water and absorbed in small intestine

VITAMIN D

RDA	5-10 ug/day for adults (10 ug equals 400 IU)
Principle sources	Sunlight, liver oils, margarine, lard, egg yolks, Vitamin D milk, shrimp, salmon, tuna
Function in body	Growth and repair of bone, maintains balance of calcium and phosphorus
Storage in body	Liver and skin
Overdose symptoms	Calcification of kidneys, blood vessels and skin, 1,000 units/lb/day in adults, kidney stones
Deficiency symptoms	Rickets, bowed legs, growth retardation, pigeon breast, osteomalacia, osteoporosis (fragile bones), increased tooth decay, decreased muscle tone
Persons at risk	Pregnancy, areas with little natural sunlight, elderly, lead posioning
Antagonists	Coristone, anticonvulsants
Synergists	Vitamin A, B_1, B_3, C and calcium
Comments	Mild bone deformities due to diet may be reversed serious deformities are permanent

VITAMIN E (TOCOPHEROL)

RDA	8-10 mg or TEs
Principle sources	Margarine, oils, chocolate, peanuts, whole grains, wheat germ, yeast, asparagus, broccoli, cabbage
Function in body	Needed for metabolism of fats. Maintains cell membrane integrity. Aids in prevention of premature aging. Aids in stress response of body. Protects against lung damage by pollutants/smoking.
Storage in body	Muscle, fatty tissue and liver in minute quantities
Overdose symptoms	Rare, may raise blood pressure
Deficiency symptoms	None found, except in low birth-weight infants who may suffer from hemolysis of RBCs
Antagonists	Rancid fats and oils, iron if taken at the same time, oral contraceptives, thyroid hormone, mineral oil
Synergists	Vitamin A, B complex, C, hormones, cortisone, testosterone, STH
Comments	Never take Vitamin E and iron together

VITAMIN K

RDA	50-60 ug
Principles sources	Green leafy vegetables, cabbage, kale, spinich, alfalfa, beef, pork, liver, cauliflower, tomatoes, carrots

Function in body	Aids in blood clotting process
Storage in body	Liver in small amounts. Vitamin K is produced daily by intestinal flora
Overdose symptoms	Not found, most likely due to limited storage
Deficiency symptoms	Rare in healthy persons. Hemorrhaging, hypoprothrombinemia or a tendency to bleed easily
Persons at risk	Newborn infants (until intestinal floras take over in first 72 hours). Chronic diarrhea, colitis or other disorders that interfere with intestinal absorption.
Antagonists	Anticoagulants, penicillin, tetracycline, sulfonamides, aspirin, mineral oil
Synergists	Vitamin A, C, E
Comments	Vitamin K IM is often given to newborns

The water soluble vitamins include all of the B complex vitamins and vitamin C. Some characteristics these vitamins share include:

- Dissolve in water
- Rapid absorption into body tissues
- Rapid excretion from body
- Need for regular dietary supplement due to rapid excretion
- Poorly stored in the body
- Excessive amounts are excreted in urine and sweat

- Tend to work together (as co-enzymes) within the body
- Easily destroyed by processing, storage, food preparation

VITAMIN B₁ (Thiamin)

RDA	1.5 mg/day
Principle sources	Brewer's yeast, wheat germ, whole grains, liver, kidney, pork, plums, prunes, raisins, sunflower seeds, nuts
Function in body	Maintains the health of nerves, heart, muscle and GI tissue, promotes growth and cell repair, needed to release energy from carbohydrates
Deficiency symptoms	Fatigue, weight loss, stomach upset, weakness, memory loss, depression, irritability, beriberi with previous symptoms plus tissue swelling, mental and motor dysfunctions
Persons at risk	Cardiac patients, alcoholics, elderly, allergies, post-surgical patients, temperature elevation
Antagonists	Emotional stress, physical stress, nitrates, baking soda, air pollution, alcohol, antibiotics
Synergists	Vitamins B_2, B_3, B_6, B_{12}, C, E, and pantothenic acid
Comments	Absorbed in the small intestine. Minimize water in preparation of foods high in B_1

VITAMIN B₂ (Riboflavin)

RDA	1.7 mg/day for adults

Principle sources	Liver, heart, kidney, milk, eggs, eggnog, broccoli, asparagus, brewer's yeast
Function in body	Needed for conversion of protein to energy. Maintenance of mucous membranes. Fetal growth and development. Regulate the synthesis of ACTH, STH, and insulin
Deficiency symptoms	Fatigue, stomach upset, anxiety, personality disturbance, high blood pressure, angular fissures and cheilosis of lips, glossitis with smooth tongue, eyes sensitive to light, watery eyes
Persons at risk	Elderly
Antagonists	Antibiotics, oral contraceptives
Synergists	Vitamins A, B_3, E
Comments	The more protein in diet the greater need for B_2. Milk in clear glass bottles has less B_2 than milk in other packaging.

VITAMIN B_3 (Niacin, Niacinamide, Nicotinic Acid, Nicotinamide)

RDA	20 mg/day for adults
Principle sources	Liver, chicken, turkey, tuna, halibut, swordfish, roasted peanuts, yeast
Function in body	Metabolism of fats, carbohydrates and proteins. Body growth rate. May reduce cholesterol and triglycerides. Regulate the synthesis of thyroxine, insulin, STH

Deficiency symptoms	Pellagra (dermatitis, dementia, diarrhea). Mild skin rash, irritability, headache, loss of memory, loss of appetite, darkening of skin.
Persons at risk	Alcoholism, diabetics, cancer, colitis
Antagonists	Emotional stress, physical stress, antibiotics
Synergists	Vitamins A, B₁, B₂, B₆, B₁₂, C, D
Comments	Peak need is between ages 15-22 years (males), 7-14 years (female). About 50% of RDA comes from typtophan being converted to B₃ by intestinal flora

VITAMIN B6 (Pyridoxine, Pyridoxal, Pyridoxamine)

RDA	2 mg/day for adults
Principal sources	Liver, meats, fish, broccoli, salmon, peanuts, walnuts, bananas, brewer's yeast, soybeans, spinach
Functions in body	Needed for metabolism of proteins and fats. Regulates synthesis of fats. Aids in synthesis of fats. Aids in formation of RBCs, bile salts. Aids in cavity prevention
Deficiency symptoms	Skin sores, depression, irritability, weight loss, convulsions, confusion, anemia
Persons at risk	Hyperactivity, anemia, use of oral contraceptives, pregnancy
Antagonists	Oral contraceptives, isoniazid, cortisone, penicillamine
Synergists	Vitamins B₁, B₂, B₃, C, magnesium

| Comments | B$_6$ first recommended for RDA in 1968. Up to 30 mg/day may be required for women who use oral contraceptives |

VITAMIN B$_{12}$ (Cobalamin, Cyanocobalamin)

RDA	6 ug/day for adults
Principle sources	Liver, kidney, crab, salmon, sardines, herring, oysters, egg yolk, milk, cheese
Function in body	Needed by all cells. Regulates the formation of RBCs. Aids in synthesis of proteins and fats
Deficiency symptoms	Pernicious anemia (weakness, fatigue, glossitis, cracked lips). Memory loss, paranoia, moodiness
Persons at risk	Vegetarians, faulty absorption of cobalamin. Lack of intrinsic factor
Antagonists	Aspirin, codeine, neomycin, oral contraceptives
Synergists	Vitamin B$_1$, folic acid, biotin, pantothenic acid, vitamin A, C, E
Comments	Vitamin actually contains an atom of cobalt

B COMPLEX (Folic Acid, Fonacin, Folate)

RDA	200 ug
Principle sources	Kidney, liver, legumes, spinach, asparagus, mushrooms, tuna, bran, yeast
Function in body	Needed by all cells. Aids in synthesis of DNA, RNA, choline. Regulates development of nerve cells (embryo/fetus). A component of genes

	and chromosomes. Natural analgesic (painkiller)
Deficiency symptoms	Macrocytic anemia, diarrhea
Persons at risk	Alcoholics, sprue, pellagra, pregnancy, intestinal disorders, oral contraceptives
Antagonists	Alcohol, emotional stress, physical stress, sulfonamides, methotrexate
Synergists	B-complex vitamins, vitamin C, hormones: testosterone, estradiol
Comments	Synthesized by intestinal bacteria in small amounts in healthy persons

B COMPLEX (Pantothenic Acid)

RDA	4-7 mg/day for adults
Principle Sources	Found in almost every food. Brewer's yeast, meats, whole-grain cereals
Function in body	Aids in synthesis of hormones acetylcholine, STH, adrenal hormones. Aids in energy release from carbohydrates, fats and proteins. Needed for the synthesis of fatty acids. Aids in preventing infection
Deficiency symptoms	Very unusual to have deficiency. Depression, fatigue, constipation, headaches
Persons at risk	Surgical patients or others with wounds. High physical or emotional stressors
Antagonists	Methylbromide (insecticide)
Synergists	B complex vitamins, A, C, E, calcium
Comments	Known as anti-stress vitamin

B COMPLEX (Biotin)

RDA	30-100 ug/day
Principle sources	Egg yolk, pork, liver, chicken, cereals, yeast, wheat, corn, milk, legumes, nuts, mushrooms
Function in body	Regulates metabolism of unsaturated fats. Needed for normal function of sweat glands, nerve tissue, blood cells, male sex glands
Deficiency symptoms	Deficiency highly unlikely
Persons at risk	None found
Antagonists	Raw egg white (greater than 24/day), antibiotics, sulfonamides
Synergists	B complex vitamins, vitamin A, D, hormone, STH
Comments	Intestinal flora synthesize biotin

VITAMIN C (Ascorbic acid)

RDA	60 mg/day for adults
Principle sources	Citrus fruits, strawberries, cantaloupe, green peppers, broccoli, brussel sprouts, parsley
Function in body	Aids in fighting infection. Aids in maintenance of blood vessel walls. Promotes the absorption of iron. Needed for formation of bone, teeth, and cartilage. Aids in metabolism of some amino acids
Deficiency symptoms	Scurvy (tenderness in calves, muscular weakness, poor appetite, bleeding

	gums, loose teeth), easy bruising, edema, poor wound healing
Persons at risk	Infants on unsupplemented formulas. High levels of physical or emotional stress. Wounds or surgical operations
Antagonists	Air pollution, smoking, alcohol, aspirin, diuretics, prednisone, indomethacin, steroids, andi-depressants, anticoagulants
Synergists	B complex, vitamin A, K, E, hormones, STH, testosterone
Comments	No evidence of cure for common cold

PREPARING MEDICATIONS FOR ADMINISTRATION

One of the most important nursing responsibilities is the administration of medications. Errors in calculation and the administration of drugs are common, but serious problems can be avoided by following these basic rules for medication administration:

- Know the hospital policy and procedure for administration of medications.
- Check the physician's order.
- Know the Five Rights: right patient, right dose, right time, right route, right medication. Another right must also be considered, the right to refuse.
- Read each label three times.
- Ask the patient if he has any allergies to medication.
- Do not allow interruptions while preparing medications.
- Do not assume that the pharmacy is always right. Always double check.
- Never administer medications that are not labeled.
- When in doubt, do not mix drugs.
- Never pour liquid back into the bottle.
- Always check the patient's armband before administering medication.
- Double check calculations.

- Insulin and heparin dosages should always be checked by a second nurse. Check PTT before giving heparin.

- Know the antidote, especially when giving IV medications.

- Know the action, side-effects, and adverse reactions of drugs before administering them.

- Always know the administration time required when administering any drugs IV push.

- When verifying a doctor's order, talk only with the doctor who wrote it.

PREVENTING MEDICATION ERRORS

- Beware of ambiguous drug names.

- Be suspicious of the use of multiple tablets. .

- Be suspicious of abrupt changes in medication orders.

- Always verify ambiguous orders with the physician.

- Always verify atypical drug orders.

- Do not accept drug nicknames. Only the generic and trade names are acceptable.

- Look up generic names when not absolutely certain.

- If the route is not specified, check with the physician.

- Do not interpret illegible handwriting, verify with the physician.

- Give special attention to multiple drug orders.

- Double check when the patient says, "These pills are different" or "I've already taken my pills."

DRUG CALCULATION FORMULAS

Surface Area Rule:

$$\text{Child Dose} = \frac{\text{Surface area (m}^2)}{1.73\text{m}^2} \times \text{Adult dose}$$

Calculating Strength of a Solution;

Solution Strength: Desired Solution:

$$\frac{x}{100} = \frac{\text{Amount of drug desired}}{\text{Amount of finished solution}}$$

Calculating Flow Rate for IV:

$$\text{Rate of Flow} = \frac{\text{Amount of fluid x Drop factor}}{\text{Running time in minutes}}$$

$$\frac{x}{1} = \frac{\text{(ml) (gtt/ml)}}{\text{min}}$$

Calculation of Medication Dosages:

Formula Method:

$$\frac{\text{Amount ordered}}{\text{Amount on hand}} \times \text{Vehicle} = \frac{\text{Number of tablets, capsules,}}{\text{or amount of liquid to be given}}$$

Vehicle is the drug form or amount of liquid containing the dosage. Amounts used in calculation by formula must be in same system.

Ratio-Proportion Method:

1 tablet: tablet in mg on hand :: x tablet order in mg

Know or have :: Want to know or order

Multiply means and extremes, divide both sides by known amount to get X. Amounts used in equation must be in same system.

Dimensional Analysis Method:

Order in mg X $\dfrac{1 \text{ tablet or capsule}}{\text{What 1 tablet or capsule is in mg}}$ = Tablets or capsules to be given

If amounts are in different systems:

Order in mg X $\dfrac{1 \text{ tablet or capsule}}{\text{What 1 tablet or capsule is in gm}}$ X $\dfrac{1 \text{ gm}}{1000 \text{ mg}}$ = Tablets or capsules to be given

INTRAVENOUS FLUID
ADMINISTRATION

IV DRUG PRECAUTIONS

- Always check precautions listed by drug manufacturer.

- Never add calcium and magnesium to other salts.

- Never mix additives with blood.

- Do not allow solutions to infuse for more than 24 hours.

- Follow manufacturer's directions regarding storage and stability.

- Never mix two IV medications in the same syringe for IV push.

- If the compatibility status of two medications is not known, flush with sterile saline between administration of the two medications.

- Always know the length of time required for administering any drug IV push.

- Always know the antidote and where to find it quickly when giving IV meds.

IV FLOW RATE CALCULATIONS
DROPS PER MINUTE

$$\frac{\text{Total ml to be infused X Drop factor*}}{\text{Total time in minutes}} = \begin{array}{l} \text{Drops / min} \\ \text{or Flow rate} \end{array}$$

INFUSION TIME

$$\frac{\text{Total ml to be infused}}{\text{ml delivered per hr.}} = \begin{array}{c}\text{Infusion Time}\\ \text{(Hour)}\end{array}$$

MILLILITERS PER HOUR

$$\frac{\text{Total Infusion Volume}}{\text{Time of infusion (hours)}} = \text{Milliliters per hour}$$

*The drop factor is the number of drops in one milliliter of solution. The drop factor is determined by the tubing manufacturer and is always on the box the tubing is packaged in.

IV SOLUTIONS

The most commonly ordered IV solutions and significant factors related to their usage are listed:

D5W--Dextrose 5% in water

Characteristics

Isotonic solution contains:
50 gm dextrose/L
170 calories/L

Indications

Emergency line assess
Fluid replacement
KVO line
Administration of IV drugs

Monitor

Increasing intracranial pressure
Fluid overload

Contraindications

>Congestive heart failure
>Increasing intracranial pressure
>Suspected head trauma
>Pulmonary edema
>Early postoperative due to increased ADH secretion
>Kidney damage
>Blood transfusions

0.9% Sodium Chloride--Normal saline

Characteristics

>Crystalloid isotonic solution contains:
>>9.0 gm NaCl/L
>>154 mEq Na/L
>>154 mEq Cl/L

Indications

>Shock, restores volume in hypovolemia
>Replaces salt
>Metabolic alkalosis
>Severe vomiting, esp. in obstruction
>Irrigation solution
>Initiate and end blood transfusion

Monitor

>Fluid overload
>Vital signs
>Breath sounds
>Intake and output
>Weight
>Hypernatremia/acidosis (with more than 1 L)
>Hypokalemia
>Lab values, esp. Na, K, Cl, bicarbonate

Contraindications
>   Congestive heart failure
>   Pulmonary edema
>   Renal dysfunction
>   Hepatic disease
>   Edema--sodium retention
>   Hypernatremia
>   Metabolic alkalosis
>   Corticosteriods
>   Debilitated or elderly
>   Mannitol administration

D5/0.2% NaCl--Dextrose 5% in water with 0.2% sodium chloride--D5 with quarter normal saline

Characteristics
>   Isotonic solution containing:
>   38.5 mEq Na/L
>   38.5 mEq Cl/L
>   50 gm dextrose/L
>   170 calories/L

Indications
>   Replacement of electrolytes
>   Calories
>   Monitor
>   Intake and output
>   Weight
>   Sodium chloride

Contraindications
>   Hypernatremia
>   Edema--sodium retention
>   Hyperglycemia
>   Delirum tremens

Hemorrhage, esp. cranial, spinal
Congestive heart failure

D5/0.45% NaCl--Dextrose 5% in water with 0.45% sodium chloride-- D5 and half-normal saline

Characteristics
Hypotonic solution contains:
50 gm dextrose/L
4.5 gm NaCl/L
77 mEq Na/L
77 mEq Cl/L
170 calories/L

Indications
Fluid maintenance
Replacement of electrolytes
Calories

Monitor
Intake and output
Weight
Sodium chloride

Contraindications
Congestive heart failure
Renal disease
Edema - sodium retention
Hypernatremia
Hyperglycemia
Delirum tremens
Hemorrhage

D5/0.9% NaCl--Dextrose 5% in water with 0.9% sodium chloride--D5 with normal saline

Characteristics

Isotonic solution containing:
154 mEq Na/L
154 mEq Cl/L
50 gm glucose/L
170 calories/L

Indications

Hydration in excess fluid loss, esp. in diaphoresis, vomiting, gastric suctioning
Replacement of electrolytes
Calories

Monitor

Intake and output
Weight daily
Breath sounds
Vital signs

Contraindications

Intracranial hemorrhage
Intraspinal hemorrhage
Delirum tremens
Diabetic coma, esp. with hyperglycemia

D5/LR--Dextrose 5% in water with lactated Ringer's solution

Characteristics

Isotonic solution containing:
130 mEq Na/L
4 mEq K/L
3 mEq Ca/L

    109 mEq Cl/L
    28 mEq lactate/L
    50 gm dextrose
    170 calories/L

Indications

    Acidosis
    Calories
    Hydration

Monitor

    Intake and output
    Weight daily
    Lab values, esp.   sodium, chloride, calcium,
       potassium

Contraindications:

    Renal disease

D5/Ringers--Dextrose 5% in water with Ringer's solution

Characteristics

    Isotonic solution containing:
        147.5 mEq Na/L
        4 mEq K/L
        4.5 meEq Ca/L
        156 mEq Cl/L
        170 calories/L

Indications

    Hydration
    Electrolyte replacement

Monitor

    Intake and output
    Weight daily
    Lab values, esp. electrolytes

Contraindications
>   Alkalosis

D10--Dextrose 10% in water

Characteristics
>   Hypertonic solution containing:
>>   100 gm dextrose/L
>>   340 calories/L

Indications
>   Hypoglycemia
>   Combined with amino acids for calories in TPN

Monitor
>   Intake and output
>   Weight daily
>   IV sites, use large veins only

Contraindications
>   Hyperglycemia
>   Delirum tremens
>   Intracranial hemorrhage
>   Congestive heart failure
>   Allergy to corn products

D50--Dextrose 50% in water

Characteristics
>   Hypertonic solution containing:
>>   500 gm dextrose/L
>>   1700 calories

Indications
>   Hypoglycemia
>   Diuresis
>   Shock

Monitor

Glucose levels
Hypokalemia
Fluid overload

Contraindications

Thrombosis
Hypokalemia
Diabetes
Corticosteriods
Do not administer with sodium bicarbonate
Do not administer with coumadin
Do not administer with whole blood

LR--Lactated Ringer's solution

Characteristics

Isotonic solution containing:
147 mEq Na/L
4 mEq K/L
4.5 mEq Ca/L
156 mEq Cl/L
28 mEq Lactate/L

Indications

Replacement solution in burns
Mild metabolic acidosis
Fluid losses, esp. GI
Hypovolemia

Monitor

Intake and output
Weight daily
Breath sounds
Vital signs
Sodium levels

Contraindications
> Anoxia
> Metabolic acidosis
> Metabolic alkalosis
> Hypernatremia
> Liver dysfunction

0.2% KCL in D5W--0.2% potassium chloride and dextrose 5% in water

Characteristics
> Isotonic solution containing:
>> 27 mEq K/L
>> 27 mEq Cl/L
>> 50 gm glucose
>> 170 calories

Indications
> Replaces KCL
> Supplies calories
> Replaces water

Monitor
> Intake and output
> K levels
> Breath sounds

Counterindications
> Hyperkalemia

ADMINISTRATION OF BLOOD AND BLOOD COMPONENTS

Blood/Blood Components	Indications For Use	Nursing Interventions
Whole Blood	Restores volume. Increases O_2 carrying capacity. Hemorrhage.	Take baseline vital signs. Type, crossmatch. Warm blood. Start at 5 ml /min. Stay with patient first 15 min. Monitor vital signs. Assess chest sounds every 15 min. Complete unit in four hours. Administer only with normal saline. Never add any medications. Use large bore needle (18-gauge).

Complications	Assessment	Interventions
Fluid overload	Distended neck veins, dyspnea, wet cough, crackles	Stop blood KVO with NS. Call physician. Fowlers' position. Notify blood bank.
Hyperkalemia	Restlessness, nausea, weakness, confusion	Assess for signs and symtoms as listed. Call physician.

Complications	Assessment	Interventions
Hypercalemia	Tingling, numbness in fingers, muscle spasm tetany.	Notify physician

Blood/Blood Components	Indications for Use	Nursing Interventions
Packed Red Blood Cells (RBCs)	Increase O_2 carrying capacity Anemia Leukemia Most used of all components because of fewer reactions.	Stay with patient 15 min. Administer slow 20-30 ml/hr in first 15 min.; then increase to 100-200 ml/hr. Normal saline may be used with RBCs. Combine no other solution and add no medication. Use blood filter.
Platelets	Increases platelets, aiding clot formation Thromocytopenia Leukemia	Infuse rapidly, in less than 30 mins. per unit.
Plasma, fresh or frozen	Expands volume Burns Trauma Various clotting factors and factor deficiencies	Check ABO compatibility. Do not heat frozen plasma. Administer within 1 hour. Never add medications.

Complications	Assessment	Interventions
Packed Red Blood Cells (RBCs): Bacterial contamination, RBC hemolysis	Febrile reaction, fever, chills, headache, tachycardia, restlessness, flushing	Stop blood. KVO with NS. Call physician. Notify blood bank. Collect urine. Draw blood according to hospital policy and send to the lab. Return to blood bank. Take vital signs every 15 mins.
Platelets: Allergic reaction	Rash Flushing Wheals Anaphylaxis Laryngeal edema	Stop blood. KVO with NS. Prepare to give Benadryl or Epinephrine as ordered.
Plasma, fresh or frozen: Hepatitis Hypocalcemia Thrombocytopenia	Electrolytes Fever Allergic Reaction	Check vital signs. Monitor lab as ordered. Monitor electrolyte imbalance.

Blood/Blood Components	Indications For Use	Nursing Interventions
Cyroprecipitate	Derivative of plasma Contains high concen-trations of Factor VIII and Fibrogen Hemophilia A	Administer at 10 ml/min. Thaw in bath of 37°C.

Blood/Blood Components	Indications For Use	Nursing Interventions
Albumin	Enhances blood volume, Trauma, hemorrhage, reduces blood viscosity	Administer 2 ml/min. Assess for increasing blood pressure, pulmonary edema, congestive heart failure.

Complications	Assessment	Interventions
Circulatory overload	Chills, fever, nausea, hemorrhage	Slow rate. Call physician, cardiac monitor, auscultate heart, breath sounds.
Septic reaction	Chills, fever, vomiting, diarrhea, hypotension	Stop infusion. KVO with NS. Obtain blood culture from donor blood and recipient. Send remaining fluid to lab.
Severe Hemolytic Reaction	Fever, chills, shock, red urine, renal failure, chest pain	Prepare to administer antibiotics, IV fluids. Verify type, cross-match. Prepare to give Lasix and insert Foley, send urine to lab.

COMPARISON OF INSULIN PREPARATIONS

Classifica-tion	Prepara-tion	Trade Name	Onset (hr)	Peak (hr)	Duration
Rapid-acting	Insulin Injection (Regular)	Regular Iletin I Actrapid Humulin/R Novolin R, Velosulin	1/2 to 1	2 to 3	5 to 7
	Prompt insulin zinc Suspension (Semilente)	Semilente Iletin I Semi-tard	1/2 to 1	4 to 7	12-16
Intermedi-ate-acting	Isophane insulin Suspension (NPH)	NPH Iletin, Humulin N, Insulatard NPH	1 to 2	8 to 12	24
	Insulin zinc suspen-sion (Lente)	Lente Iletin I, Lentard Monotard	1 to 2	8 to 12	24
Long-acting	Extended insulin zinc suspension	Ultralente Iletin Ultratard	4 to 8	16 to 18	36

HOW TO CHOOSE ROTATION SITES

These areas of the body are most commonly recommended as rotation sites when administering insulin. The rotation aids in absorption as well as preventing buildup of hardened tissue. Choose one of these sites on a rotating basis:

- Outer area of the upper arm
- Just above and below the waist, except for within a 2-inch radius of the navel
- Upper area of the buttock, just behind the hip bone
- Front of the thigh, to about 4 inches above the knee

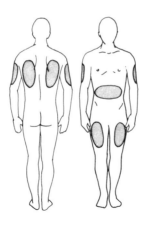

DRUG INCOMPATIBILITY CHART

CLASSIFICATION   POTENTIAL INCOMPATIBILITIES

Analgesic Drugs

Aspirin (salisylate)
Dololid
Ibuprofen
Indocin
Narcotics: codeine,
morphine, demerol

Anticoagulants: GI bleeding, especially
with aspirin. Corticosteroids: Decreases
analgesic effects, increases GI irritation.
Sulfonylureas: Large doses of aspirin
potentiates antidiabetics. Diuretics:
Decreases action of spironolactone. Anticonvulsants: Potentiates phenytoin. Alcohol (at high levels): Respiratory
depression, hypotension, coma.

Antiarrhythmic Drugs

Bretylium (emergency)
Lidocaine (emergency)
Nitroglycerin
Quinidine
Verapamil

Anticoagulants: Increased bleeding time.
Antihypertensives: Hypotension.
Muscle relaxants: Potentiates, action of
relaxants.
Cholinergic agents: Antagonism of
cholinergic effects.
MAOI: Do not take with propranolol.

Antihypertensive Drugs

Aldomet
Apresoline
Capoten
Catapres
Corgard
Diazoxide (emergency)
Hyperstat (emergency)
Inderal
Lopresor
Minipress

Antidepressants: Increased hypertension.
CNS depressant: Enhanced depressive ef-
fect on CNS.
Diuretics: Hyperglycemia, enhances an-
tihypertensive effects.
Alcohol: Orthostatic hypotension.
Digitalis: Bradycardia.
Inderal: Hypotension.

CLASSIFICATION   POTENTIAL INCOMPATIBILITIES

Antimicrobial Drugs

Acyclovir
Amoxicillin
Ampicillin
Cephalosporins
Erythromycin
Gentamycin
Griseofulvin
Neomycin
Penicillins

Penicillin concentrations: Aspirin and
probenicid.
Anticoagulants: Increased bleeding time.
Antacids: Decreases absorption, especially with tetracycline.

Anticoagulant Drugs

Heparin
Coumadin

Many medications increase anticoagula-
tion activity when used in conjunction
with anticoagulants. Among them:

> Alcohol
>
> Antibiotics
>
> Aspirin
>
> Chloral hydrate
>
> Diazoxide
>
> Dilantin
>
> Persantine
>
> Thyroid hormones
>
> Zyloprim

Medications that decrease anticoagu-
lant activity are:

> Aldactone
>
> Barbiturates
>
> Tegretol
>
> Vitamin K

CLASSIFICATION	POTENTIAL INCOMPATIBILITIES

Cardiovascular Drugs

Digitoxin
Digoxin
Dopamine
  (emergency)
Epinephrine
  (emergency)
Nitroglycerin

Antifungals: Hypokalemia and digitalis toxicity.
Antacids: Inhibits digitalis action.
Verapamil: Bradycardia.
Corticosteroids: Hypokalemia and digitalis toxicity.
Diuretics: Hypomagnesemia and hypokalemia with digitalis toxicity.

Diuretic Drugs

Aldactone
Lasix
Mannitol
HCTZ
Dyazide

Anticoagulants: Increased bleeding time.
Antidiabetics: Hyperglycemia.
Antihypertensives: Hypotension.
Corticosteroids: Potassium loss.
Lithium: Elevated lithium levels.
MAOI: Hypotension.
Muscle relaxants: Increased action by both drugs.
Aspirin: Salicylate toxicity with large doses.
Digitalis: Potassium loss.

Alcohol

Any product containing alcohol.

Anticoagulants: Inhibited with chronic use; accentuated with high alcohol blood levels. Antihistamines: CNS depression. Aspirin: GI bleeding. Barbiturates: Decreased in chronic use; potentiated in high alcohol levels. Hypoglycemics: Hypoglycemia more pronounced. Antabuse: Hyperventilation, hypotension, death. MAOI: Sedation, hypertensive crisis. Tricyclic antidepressants: CNS depression, sedation.

CLASSIFICATION   POTENTIAL INCOMPATIBILITIES

Sedative-Hypnotic Drugs

Chloral hydrate
Dalmane
Halcion
Phenobarbital
Restoril
Seconal

Alcohol: CNS depression. Anticonvulsants: Increases effect of drugs such as Dilantin. Anticoagulants: Increased bleeding time. Antidepressants: Enhances depression, transient delirium with Elavil. Corticosteroids: Decreased action of steroids. MAOI: Potentiates actions of barbiturates.

Oral Contraceptive Drugs

Enviod
Lo/Ovral
Norinyl
Ortho-Novum
Ovcon

Anticoagulants: Decreases effectiveness of anticoagulants. Anticonvulsants: Dilantin toxicity. Breakthrough bleeding which indicates decreased effectiveness of contraceptive control. Barbiturates: Breakthrough bleeding with decrease in contraceptive effectiveness. Antibiotics: Breakthrough bleeding and decreased control.

GUIDE TO AVOIDING DRUG INCOMPATIBILITIES/INTERACTIONS

The highest potential of drug incompatibility exists when:

- More than one drug is added to a solution such as IV fluids.

- IV solutions and medications are administered via the same IV line.

- A medication is reconstituted with the wrong solution.

- Any solution is mixed with diazepam (Valium).

- Any solution is mixed with diphenylhydantoin (Dilantin).

- Sodium bicarbonate is administered with epinephrine. The IV line should be flushed.

- Penicillins are mixed with ascorbic acid or tetracycline.

- Reconstituted medications are kept at the wrong temperature. Most need to be refrigerated.

- More than one antibiotic is administered at a time. The IV line should be flushed and administration times are staggered when possible.

Controlled substance chart

Drugs	United States	Canada
Heroin, LSD, peyote, marijuana, mescaline	Schedule I	Schedule H
Opium, morphine, meperidine, amphetamines, cocaine, short-acting barbiturates (secobarbital)	Schedule II	Schedule G
Glutethimide Paregoric, phen-dimetrazine	Schedule III	Schedule F
Chloral hydrate, chlor-diazepoxide, diazepam, mazin-dol, meprobamate, phenobarbital	Schedule IV	Schedule F
Antidiarrheals with opium, antitussives	Schedule V	

FDA Pregnancy Categories

A   No risk demonstrated to the fetus in any trimester

B   No adverse effects in animals, no human studies available

C   Only given after risks to the fetus are considered: animal studies have shown adverse reactions, no human studies available

D   Definite fetal risks, may be given in spite of risks if needed in life-threatening conditions

X   Absolute fetal abnormalities; not to be used anytime in pregnancy

Immunization Table

Age	0.5 ML IM	0.5 ML SC
2 mo	DPT, HbOC	OPV
4 mo	DPT, HbOC	OPV
6 mo	DPT, HbOC	OPV
15 mo	MMR	
18 mo	DPT	OPV (Polio)
4-6 yr	DPT	OPV (Polio)
11-12 yr	MMR	
14-16 yr	Td*	

*Tetanus toxoid. Repeat every 10 years

CONTRAINDICATIONS:

Leukemia	Blood transfusion within 3 mo.	Steroid therapy
Malignancy	Immunoglogulin within 3 mo.	Hypersensitivity
Lymphoma	Maternal antibodies within 3 mo.	Radiation therapy
Chemotherapy	Pregnancy for MMR only	

Body Surface Area Method

LaRocca and Otto give the formula and nomogram for determining dosage for a child based on height, weight, and body surface area (Fig 24-1). Height is correlated with the weight of the child to determine the body surface area of the child. The drug dose is then ordered as mg/m2.

Plot the height and weight of the child on the nomogram (which is a graphic representation of a numeric relationship) to determine the body surface are (BSA). Multiply the BSA (which is given in square meters on the nomogram) by mg/m2.

Example: The drug literature recommends 1 mg/m2.

0.50 x 1 mg = x dose

x = 0.50 mg of drug

Body surface area of children: nomogram for determination of body surface from height and mass, based on the formula of DuBois and DuBois.

Nomogram

Place a straight edge from the patient's height in the left column to his weight in the right column. The point of intersection on the body surface area column indicates the body surface area (BSA). Reproduced from Behrman, R.E., and Vaughn, V.C. (editors): Nelson's textbook of pediatrics, ed. 12, Philadelphia, 1983, W.B. Saunders Co.

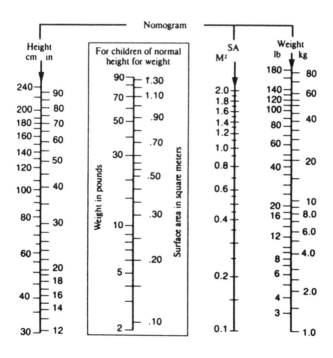

CLINICAL
SKILLS

CLINICAL SKILLS

Table of Contents

CARDIOPULMONARY RESUSCITATION

ONE RESCUER CPR; ADULT

ASSESSMENT

ACTION

1. Airway. Determine unresponsiveness. Call for help. Position victim. Open airway.

Shake shoulder, "Are you ok?" Call out, "Help!" Turn to supine position. Use head-tilt/chin-lift maneuver.

2. Breathing. Determine breathlessness. Ventilate.

Ear over mouth, observe chest: Look, listen. Feel for breathing (3-5 seconds). Seal mouth and nose. Ventilate 2 times at a rate of 1-1.5 seconds per inspiration. Watch chest rise for adequate ventilation.

3. Circulation. Determine pulselessness. Activate EMS. Begin chest compressions.

Check carotid 5-10 seconds. Maintain head tilt. If someone has responded, send them for help. Check landmark for hand placement two fingers above xyphoid process. Compress 1 1/2-2". Compression rate : 80-100 min.

4. Compression-Ventilation Ratio

15-2. 15 compressions and 2 ventilations. Do 4 cycles and check carotid (5 seconds). If no pulse, continue CPR.

TWO RESCUER CPR; ADULT

ASSESSMENT	ACTION
1. Airway (Same procedure as one man.)	
2. Breathing (Same procedure as one man.)	
3. Circulation Determine pulselessness. Compressor gets into position.	Say "No pulse." Check landmark.
4. Compression / Ventilation Ratio	Ratio: 5-1. Rate: 80-100 /min. Say any mnemonic. Stop compression to allow for each ventilation. Ventilator ventilates after every 5 compressions. After 10 cycles, ventilator checks carotid pulse.
5. Call for switch.	Compressor calls for switch. Compressor completes 5th compression. Ventilator completes ventilation, then switches.
6. Switch.	Ventilator moves to chest and compressor moves to head in simultaneous movement. New ventilator checks carotid. Say, "No pulse." Ventilate once. Continue CPR.

ONE RESCUER CPR; INFANT

ASSESSMENT	ACTION
1. Airway. (Same procedure as one man adult.)	Be careful not to hyperextend the head. Ventilate twice.
2. Breathing. (Same procedure as one man adult.)	**EXCEPTION**: Make tight seal around nose and mouth.
3. Circulation. Determine pulselessness. Activate EMS. Begin chest compression.	Feel for brachial pulse for 5-10 seconds. Draw imaginary line between nipples. Place 2-3 fingers on sternum, 1 finger's width below imaginary line. Compress vertically, 1/2-1". Say any helpful mnenonic. Compression rate: 100/min.
4. Compression/ Ventilation Ratio	Ratio: 5-1. 5 compressions to 1 slow ventilation. Pause for ventilation. Do ten cycles, then check brachial pulse. No pulse: Ventilate once. Continue CPR.

CHOKING (with CPR and ACLS)

The following sequence is recommended by the American Heart Association for the choking patient with an airway obstruction:

CONSCIOUS PATIENT WITHOUT TRAUMA

Assess obstruction by asking patient to speak. If he cannot speak or he exhibits the universal sign of grabbing throat:

Administer sub-diaphramatic abdominal thrust (also known as Heimlich maneuver). Then perform finger sweep.

Repeat this sequence until airway is clear or patient becomes unconscious.

UNCONSCIOUS PATIENT WITHOUT TRAUMA

Call for help, if possible, activating EMS system.

Open airway, if possible, providing positive pressure ventilation.

Perform finger sweep in side-lying position.

Administer 6-10 abdominal manual thrusts.

Finger sweep.

Reopen airway, reposition head, and ventilate.

Repeat this sequence until obstruction is cleared.

For pregnant women or obese people perform chest thrust only. (Do not perform abdominal thrusts).

---

*The American Heart Association is planning changes in this protocol. However, possible changes were not available at the time of publication.

CARDIAC MONITORING

Cardiac monitoring provides a continuous reading of a patient's heartbeat. Every heartbeat exemplifies a complex conduction system that is stimulated by an electrical impluse. Each beat can be monitored on an oscilloscope in a definitive pattern called an electrocardiogram (EKG or ECG).

The ECG strip is utilized to detect changes in beat and rhythm. Therefore, it is essential for the nurse to recognize the most common pathologic ECG changes.

HOW THE CONDUCTION SYSTEM WORKS

The sinoatrial (SA) node fires the first electrical impulse and rapidly discharges at 60-100 impulses per minute. The discharge pulses through the right and left atria on its way to the atrioventricular (AV) node. After a brief pause at the AV node, it travels to the Bundle of His, the right and left bundle branches, and Purkinje fibers. Then, the entire ventricular myocardium is activated.

THE ECG COMPLEX

The ECG is easily recognized on a rhythm strip. The following is a brief summary of each wave:

P WAVE--Electrical impulse firing at the SA node and traveling through the atria. This is atrial depolarization.

QRS COMPLEX--Impulse pulses down AV node, Bundle of His and bundle branches. This is ventricular depolarization.

T WAVE--Ventricular repolarization.

PR INTERVAL - Measured from beginning of P wave to beginning of Q wave. This interval of 0.12 to 0.20 second is the time it takes the impulse to reach the ventricles.

QRS INTERVAL--Measured from beginning of Q wave to the end of S wave. Represents time it takes for impulse to spread through ventricular myocardium. Duration: 0.06 to 0.1 second.

QT INTERVAL--Measured from beginning of Q wave to end of T wave. Represents total duration of ventricular contraction or systole. Its average time is 0.40 second.

THE WAVES ON AN ECG RHYTHM STRIP

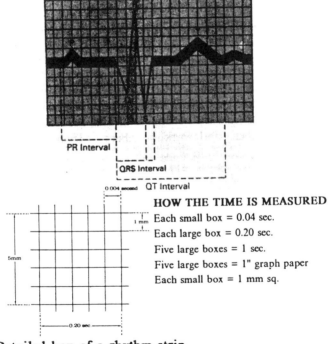

PR Interval

QRS Interval

QT Interval

0.004 second

HOW THE TIME IS MEASURED

Each small box = 0.04 sec.

Each large box = 0.20 sec.

Five large boxes = 1 sec.

Five large boxes = 1" graph paper

Each small box = 1 mm sq.

1 mm

5mm

0.20 sec

Detailed box of a rhythm strip

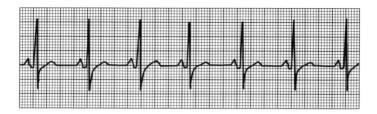

In **NORMAL SINUS RHYTHM** the rate is 60 to 100 beats/minute, rhythm is regular, P waves are present. QRS is of normal duration, P/QRS relationship and the PR interval is within normal limits.

15 large boxes = 3 seconds

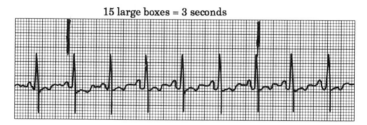

This rhythm strip can be used to calculate heart rate.

There are two methods:

If the rhythm is regular: Count the number of large boxes between the two R waves and divide the number into 300. For example, 1 box equals 300, 2 boxes equals 150 and 3 boxes equals 75.

If the rhythm is irregular: Count the number of cycles in a 6-second strip and multiply by 10. The graph paper is marked along the top in 3-second intervals.

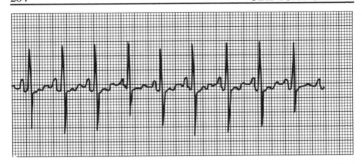

SINUS TACHYCARDIA is a heart rate over 100 beats/min.   Otherwise, the strip indicates normal sinus rhythm because there is a P wave, QRS complex, PR interval, and a T wave. Pain, smoking, congestive heart failure, high fever, anxiety, hypoxia, exercise, heart failure (early stages) and certain drugs can cause sinus tachycardia.   The underlying cause must be determined by the physician before treatment.   The underlying cause must be detected and treated. If CHF is the cause, the drug of choice is then, of course, digitalis.

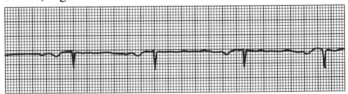

SINUS BRADYCARDIA is a heart rate less than 60 beats/min. Bradycardia is considered normal in athletes who undergo intense physical conditioning. It is seen abnormally in   hyperkalemia,   myocardial   infarction,   increasing intracranial pressure, and   imbalance of certain drugs such as digitalis and Inderal.   Atropine or Isuprel IV is administered to increase heart rate. A pacemaker may be indicated if the patient develops severe hypotension, syncope, or acidosis.

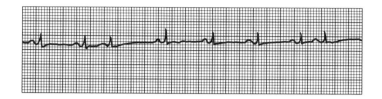

This strip shows **PREMATURE ATRIAL CONTRACTIONS (PACs)**. The P waves vary in shape and location because the stimulation does not originate in the SA node. The rate is 60-100 beats/minute and the rhythm is irregular. Fatigue, smoking, alcohol, caffeine, and ischemia are among the possible causes of PACs. If more than six PACs per minute occur, oxygen should be administered. Medications to follow may include quinidine, procainamide, or digitalis.

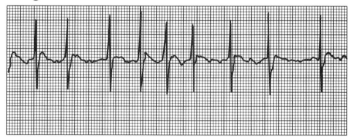

This wavy, irregular baseline is **ATRIAL FIBRILLATION**. In atrial fibrillation the SA node is firing impulses at a very fast pace--up to 400/minute. The AV node picks up the impulses at random and produces irregular ventricular contractions. This results in decreased cardiac output, congestive heart failure, and/or shock because the atria never fully contact. Atrial fibrillation is treated with digoxin and Verapamil IV, or digitalis orally.

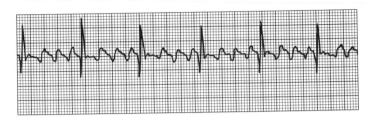

   This sawtooth pattern is typical of **ATRIAL FLUTTER**
and can go as high as 240-360 beats/minute. The sawtooth
pattern is created by very rapid firing in the atria, so that
only about one in four impulses actually reach the ventricle.
Even then, ventricle response will vary and the PR interval
will be irregular, causing the sawtooth pattern. Atrial flutter
is   potentially   dangerous   because   ineffective   atrial
contractions can cause clots that break away and become
emboli.   Flutter is less common than atrial fibrillation, but
the complications and results are much the same.   Atrial
flutter is most commonly seen in patients with coronary
artery disease or rheumatic heart disease.   Treatment is
initally digitalis, followed by quinidine. Procainamide and
propranolol also may be ordered.

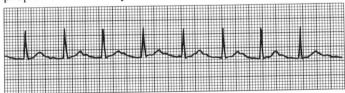

   Abnormally long PR intervals are characteristic of
FIRST DEGREE AV BLOCK.   The rate is 60-100
beats/minute. The impulse originates in the SA node, but
runs into a block at the AV node. Treatment is aimed at the
underlying cause.   Causes include anoxia, myocardial
ischemia, AV node malfunction, myocarditis, and drugs such
as digitalis, clonidine, and tricyclic antidepressants.   If

digitalis toxicity is suspected, withhold drug until a serum level can be drawn. In the meantime, administer oxygen. If patient experiences pain, syncope, or bradycardia, atropine is administered. If patient is unresponsive to atropine, isoproterenol may be given IV. If drug therapy is unsuccessful, prepare patient for a pacemaker.

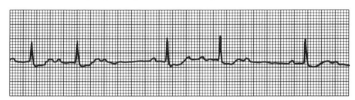

SECOND-DEGREE AV BLOCK is also called Wenckebach or Mobitz I. The atrial rate is 60-100 beats/min, but the lack of ventricular stimulation usually leads to bradycardia. This block is often the result of an anterior MI. Other causes include digitalis toxicity or hyperkalemia. Drug therapy includes digitalis, and if unsuccessful, followed by isoproterenol. If digitalis is the cause, draw a serum level and administer O_2. If hyperkalemia is the cause, prepare to administer a Kay-exalate enema. This patient may need a pacemaker.

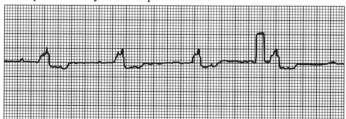

SECOND-DEGREE AV BLOCK or **MOBITZ II**, is basically the same as Wenckebach, with slow ventricular stimulation and bradycardia. Atropine is indicated.

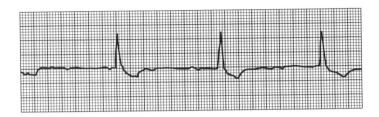

THIRD-DEGREE AV BLOCK (Stokes-Adams Syndrome) is an atrial rate of 60-100 beats/minute with complete ventricular asystole. This means the SA node is sending the impulse, but it is blocked at the AV node. The ventricles do not contract, therefore, there are no QRS complexes or PR intervals; only continuous P waves. There is no cardiac output during a third-degree block. Drug therapy is isoproterenol followed by insertion of a pacemaker. The physician may consider an atropine bolus before starting isoproterenol drip.

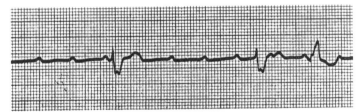

THIRD DEGREE BLOCK, or **COMPLETE HEART BLOCK,** occurs when the impulse from the SA node is completely blocked. The ventricles begin to initiate impulses and beat on their own. The atria and ventricles are beating independently of each other. Causes include MI and digitalis toxicity. Atropine or isoproterenol may be given initially, followed by a pacemaker.

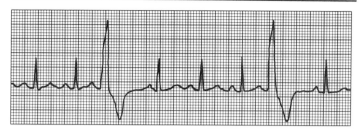

PREMATURE VENTRICULAR CONTRACTIONS

occur when the ventricles are irritated enough to initiate a ventricular beat. This "extra beat" is seen in a wide and rather bizarre QRS complex. PVCs are rather common, and the cause can be widely varied, including hypoxia, ischemia, MI, hyperkalemia, use of alcohol, drugs, and caffeine. In the elderly, PVCs often occur without pathology, and the administration of oxygen will allieviate the impulse. PVCs occur in patterns. Bigeminy is a PVC every other beat, trigeminy is a PVC every third beat, couplets are a pair of PVCs, and a triplet is three at a time. A series of 6 or more is ventricular tachycardia. The focus of therapy is to treat the underlying cause. If the cause cannot be immediately determined, give lidocaine bolus followed by an IV drip. The physician may also consider atropine, procainamide, quinidine, phenytoin, bretylium, or propranolol.

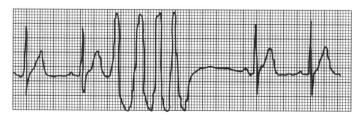

This is ventricular tachycardia of three or more PVCs are followed by normal sinus rhythm.   Lidocaine is indicated.

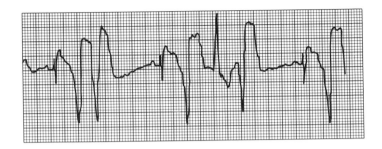

MULTIFOCAL PREMATURE VENTRICULAR CONTRACTIONS (PVCs) are more dangerous than occasional, unifocal beats. More than three sustained PVCs results in ventricular tachycardia.

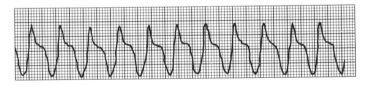

VENTRICULAR TACHYCARDIA can hit 200 beats/minute and is a dangerous condition. Lidocaine IVP will be ordered. If V tach is not halted, it will deteriorate to ventricular fibrillation. Cardiac arrest will soon follow. Defibrillation will be utilized if there are no impulses present. If defibrillator is not available, perform CPR. If defibrillation is unsuccessful, prepare to administer epinephrine, lidociane, and bretylium, alternating with defibrillation.

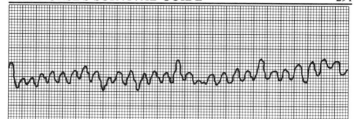

VENTRICULAR FIBRILLATION is indicated by this chaotic line. The rate is rapid and disorganized, the rhythm irregular, and the ventricles are firing so fast that a quivering line takes the place of P waves, QRS complexes, and PR intervals. It is the most common strip seen in cardiac arrest. There is no cardiac output, and death will result in less than six minutes if this fibrillation persists. Physician will follow ACLS guidelines in administering medications and defibrillation.

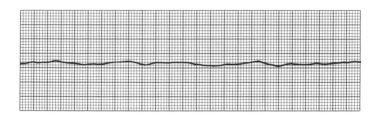

ASYSTOLE OR VENTRICULAR STANDSTILL indicates that cardiac arrest has occurred and has been sustained, unresponsive to treatment. The patient's heart has stopped functioning. CPR and ACLS will be initiated. Mortality is greater than 95%. The physician may defribillate, administer epinephrine, atropine, and may consider sodium bicarbonate for acidosis. (Note: Always check the leads first, this straight line could be caused by an interrupted connection.)

ADVANCED CARDIAC LIFE SUPPORT (ACLS)

Advanced cardiac life support (ACLS) utilizes advanced airway management, defibrillation, emergency medications, and basic CPR. Most cardiac arrests are related to ventricular fibrillation and are not witnessed. The following is the basic protocol for an adult with an unwitnessed cardiac arrest associated with ventricular fibrillation and/or pulseless ventricular tachycardia.

1. Check pulse, if absent, procede as follows.
2. Perform CPR until defibrillator is available. Then apply paste on the right upper sternum and one at the left axillary line. Attach paddles as directed.
3. Check rhythm. If ventricular fibrillation or ventricular tachycardia appears, procede.
4. Defibrillate at 200 joules. If no conversion, continue.
5. Defibrillate at 200-300 joules. If no conversion, continue.
6. Defibrillate at full output, 360 joules.
7. Continue with CPR if no pulse.
8. Establish IV line.
9. Administer epinephrine 1:10,000 solution 0.5-1.0 mg IV push.
10. Intubate.
11. Defibrillate at 360 joules. If no conversion, continue.
12. Administer lidocaine 1 mg/kg IV push.
13. Defibrillate with 360 joules. If no conversion, continue.
14. Repeat lidocaine 0.5 mg/kg IV push. Administer up to 3.0 mg/kg total lidocaine. Repeat boluses of 0.5 mg/kg at 8-minute intervals.
15. Defibrillate at 360 joules. If no conversion, continue.

16. Administer bretylium 5 mg/kg IV push.
17. Consider bicarbonate.
18. Defibrillate at 360 joules.
19. Repeat lidocaine or bretylium.
20. Defibrillate at 360 joules.

RESUSCITATION DRUGS

DRUG	ADULT DOSE	PEDIATRIC DOSE
Atropine	Asystole: 1 mg IV, repeat in 5 min; bradycardia: 0.5 mg IV q 5 min until 2 mg is administered	0.01-0.03 mg/kg IV
	INDICATIONS	**CONSIDERATIONS**
	AV block, asystole, sinus bradycardia	After total of 2 mg administered with no response, give isoproterenol. Do not give if heart rate is over 60.
	ADULT DOSE	**PEDIATRIC DOSE**
Bretylium tosylate	Ventricular fibrillation: 5 mg/kg (350-500 mg) initial dose, followed by boluses at 10 mg/kg Ventricular	5 mg/kg, followed by boluses at 10 mg/kg

tachycardia:
500 mg in 50
ml IV solution
administered 1
mg/kg/min

INDICATIONS	CONSIDERATIONS
Recurrent ventricular tachycardia, ventricular fibrillation	After loading dose, infuse at 1-2 mg/min

DRUG	ADULT DOSE	PEDIATRIC DOSE
Calcium chloride	5-7 mg/kg IV q 10 min	0.3 ml/kg IV (10% solution)

INDICATIONS	CONSIDERATIONS
Hypocalcemia, hyperkalemia	Flush line before administering sodium bicarbonate. Often used in dialysis patients and in calcium channel blocker overdose.

DRUG	ADULT DOSE	PEDIATRIC DOSE
Dopamine (Intropin)	2.5-10 ug/kg/min, titrate to effect	Same as adult

INDICATIONS	CONSIDERATIONS
Cardiogenic, septic shock	Increases renal flow, monitor closely as effects vary

DRUG	ADULT DOSE	PEDIATRIC DOSE
Epinephrine (Adrenaline)	0.5-1.0 mg IV every 5 minutes during cardiac arrest (5-10 ml of 1:10,000 solution). Can be administered endotracheal route	0.1 ml/kg IV q 5 min (1:10,000 solution)
	INDICATIONS	**CONSIDERATIONS**
	First line drug in V fib and pulseless V tach; Asystole, ventricular fibrillation	Flush line before adminstering sodium bicarb. Can be given through ET tube
DRUG	**ADULT DOSE**	**PEDIATRIC DOSE**
Isoproterenol (Isuprel)	2-10 ug/min IV, titrate to effect	Start 0.1 ug/kg/min, titrate to effect
	INDICATIONS	**CONSIDERATIONS**
	Bradycardia Bronchospasm, Heart block, Ventricular deprhythmias, Shock	Contraindicated in tachycardia and recent MI. Use cautiously in diabetes. Closely monitor diastolic, as it may drop marketdly
DRUG	**ADULT DOSE**	**PEDIATRIC DOSE**
Lidocaine (Xylocaine)	1 mg/kg IV bolus, then 0.5 mg.kg q 8-10 min to total 3 mg/kg	1 mg/kg/dose IV, then 30 ug/kg/min drip

	INDICATIONS	**CONSIDERATIONS**
	PVCs, tachycardia, ventricular fibrillation	Administer drip after bolus to maintain effect (adult 2-4 mg/kg)
DRUG	**ADULT DOSE**	**PEDIATRIC DOSE**
Sodium Bicarbonate	1 mEq/kg IV, then 1/2 dose q 10 min. Draw ABGs to consider further dosages	1-2 mEq/kg IV, then 1 mEq q 10 min
	INDICATIONS	**CONSIDERATIONS**
	Hyperkalemia, severe acidosis during MI	Flush line before administering calcium or epinephrine. No longer recommended for routine use in MI, only for "consideration"
DRUG	**ADULT DOSE**	**PEDIATRIC DOSE**
Verapamil (Isoptin)	5 mg IV, 10 mg in 15 min if dysrhythmia persists	0.1-0.3 mg/kg IV, repeat dose in 30 min, if needed, 0.1-0.2 mg/kg
	INDICATIONS	**CONSIDERATIONS**
	Supraventricular tachycardia, atrial fibrillation or flutter	Administer slowly over 1 minute (3 minutes in the elderly); use carotid massage before verapamil. May decrease arterial pressure, may worsen CHF

	ADULT DOSE	**PEDIATRIC DOSE**
Defibrillation	200-300 joules repeat X1, then full output if required.	2 joules/kg, advance to 6 joules/kg maximum

	INDICATIONS	**CONSIDERATIONS**
	Ventricular fibrillation, pulseless ventricular tachycardia	Synchronizer OFF or unit may not fire

OTHER COMMONLY-USED
EMERGENCY MEDICATIONS

Digoxin

(Lanoxin)

Indications in Emergencies:

Congestive heart failure

Cardiogenic shock

Atrial fibrillation

Administer:

Adult: 0.5 to 1 mg IV or PO as initial dose;
0.25 to 0.5 mg for maintenance

Pediatric: Dosages vary with age, consult product
information

Nursing Implications:

Do not give in conjunction with calcium chloride

Do not give in hyperkalemia or hypokalemia

Increases AV conduction time

Do not give in heart block

Use cautionally with Dilantin and epinephrine

Furosemide

(Lasix)

Indications in Emergencies:

Congestive heart failure

Pulmonary edema

Cerebral edema (in head injuries)

Administer:

Adult: 20-40 mg IV bolus slowly (over 2-4 minutes)

Pediatric: 1-2 mg/kg IV, not to exceed 6 mg/kg/24 hr

Nursing Implications:

Strict I&O, especially urinary output;

> Monitor for hypovolemia as diuresis may cause sudden volume depletion
>
> Do not give in pregnancy

Morphine Sulfate

Indications in Emergencies:

> Severe pain: renal colic and burns
>
> Drug of choice in pain of myocardial infarction
>
> Pulmonary edema to decrease venous return to right side of heart

Administer:

> Adult: 2-15 mg IV, slowly
>
> Pediatric: 0.1 to 0.2 mg/kg IV slowly titrated

Nursing Implications:

> Monitor respiratory rate; can cause respiratory depression if given too quickly
>
> Have 0.5 mg narcan ready as a antidote
>
> Do not give if head trauma is suspected
>
> Can be addictive

Naloxone

(Narcan)

Indications in Emergencies:

> Reverses narcotic overdose
>
> Reverses Darvon overdose
>
> Septic shock

Administer:

> Adult: 0.4-0.8 mg IV, can be administered endotracheally or sublingally
>
> Pediatric: 0.01 mg/kg IV

Nursing Implications:

> Can be used in a larger dose if necessary
>
> Will cause withdrawal symptoms in narcotic overdose

Procainamide

(Pronestyl)
Indications in Emergencies:
    Ventricular dysrhythmias
    Paroxysmal atrial tachycardia
    Atrial fibrillation
    Premature ventricular contractions
Administer:
    Adult: 100 mg slow IV push, can repeat in 3-5 minutes, not to exceed 1 gm IV drip: 1 gm in 500 ml D5W at 1-3 ml/min
    Pediatric: 2mg/kg IV bolus over 4 minutes IV drip: 10-100 mg in 500 ml D5W titrated

Nursing Implications:

    Contraindicated in heart block
    Slows heart rate and conduction system
    Watch for hallucinations

Propranolol

(Inderal)
Indications in Emergenices:
    Acute MI, especially in dysrhythmias not responsive to other cardiac drugs
    Digitalis toxicity
Administer:
    Adult: 1 mg IV, repeat 2-3 minutes; not to exceed 3 mg
    Pediatrics: Not recommended
Nursing Implications:
    Monitor for respiratory problems
    Assess for bronchoconstriction

Aminophylline

Indications in Emergencies:
    Asthma attacks
    Bronchospasm
    Pulmonary edema
    COPD
Administer:
    Adult: 250-500 mg in 20-30 ml D5W to infuse over 30 min.
    Pediatric: 4 mg/kg via IV infusion
Nursing Implications:
    Administer slowly
    Assess for restlessness, hypotension, dsyrhythmias

Cefazolin Sodium

(Ancef, Kefzol)
Indications in Emergencies:
    Severe infections, especially if cause is unknown
    Prophylactic in multiple trauma
Administer:
    Adult: 250 mg to 1 gm IV up to 6 gm in 24 hours
    Pediatric: 25-50 mg/kg q 6 hrs over 24-hour period. Contraindicated under 1 month of age
Nursing Implications:
    Monitor closely for allergic reaction and anaphylaxis.
    Contraindicated with Pronestyl, quinidine, Phenergan, and most diuretics

Cephalothin Sodium

(Keflin)
Indications in Emergencies:
    Serious infections
    Prophylactic in multiple trauma

Administer:
> Adult: 1 to 2 gm IV every 6 hours; up to 12 gm
> Pediatric: 40-80 mg/kg IV divided doses over 24 hours

Nursing Implications:
> Anaphylaxis common
> Incompatible with many other medications

Chloramphenicol sodium succinate

(Chloromycetin)

Indications in Emergencies:
> Meningitis
> Rocky Mountain Spotted Fever
> Salmonella

Administer:
> Adult: 50 mg/kg/24 hours IV in 4 divided doses
> Pediatric: 25 mg/kg/24 hours in 4 divided doses

Nursing Implications:
> Given IV only, administer with extreme caution

Chlordiazepoxide hydrochloride

(Librium)

Indications in Emergencies:
> Severe anxiety and agitation
> Acute alcohol withdrawal

Administer:
> Adult: 50-100 mg po; repeat every 2 to 4 hours
> Pediatric: Not recommended

Nursing Implications:
> May be given PO, IV, IM
> PO route is preferred
> Can be addictive
> Monitor for hypotension

Dexamethasone sodium phosphate

(Decadron, Betamethasone)
Indications in Emergencies:
Shock
Allergic reactions
Cerebral edema
Acute, severe inflammations
Administer:
Adults: Doses vary widely; consult product
information
Pediatrics: Also variable
Nursing Implications:
Contraindicated in pregnancy
Can mask signs of other infections
Contraindicated in diabetes, renal disease
Observe for hypertension, hyperglycemia, euphoria

Dextrose 50%

(Glucose 50%)
Indications in Emergencies:
Hypoglycemia
When cause of coma is unknown
Administer:
Adult: 50 ml of 50% solution IV
Pediatric: 1 mg/kg of 50% solution IV
Nursing Implications:
Have serum glucose drawn before and during
administration
Thiamin 100 mg IV if alcoholism is suspected to
prevent Wernicke-Korsakoff syndrome

Diazepam

(Valium)
Indications in Emergencies:

Status epilepticus

Acute psychological distress

Prior to cardioversion

Prior to manual traction joint dislocation

Administer:

Adults: 2 to 10 mg slow IV push

Pediatrics: Not recommended

Nursing Implications:

Do not mix with any other medication when administering IV

Give slowly; it can cause respiratory depression

Monitor for confusion, syncope

Diazoxide

(Hyperstat)

Indications in Emergencies:

Malignant hypertension

Hypoglycemia

Administer:

Adult: 30 mg IV push, administered rapidly, can be repeated in 30 minutes

Pediatric: 5 mg/kg IV push

Nursing Implications:

Place patient in supine position

Check blood pressure frequently

Get baseline before administering

Watch for seizures, hyperglycemia

Diphenhydramine hydrochloride

(Benadryl)

Indications in Emergencies:

Allergic reactions

Nausea, vomiting

Phenothiazine side effects

Administer:
>   Adult: 10 to 50 mg IV over 4 min
>   Pediatric: 2 mg/kg IV over 1-4 min

Nursing Implications:
>   Caution patient it may cause drowsiness
>   Do not give if patient is hypertensive
>   Do not give if patient has history of glaucoma

Heparin

Indications in Emergencies:
>   Auto transfusions
>   Disseminated intravascular coagulation (DIC)
>   Pulmonary embolism
>   Atrial fibrillation
>   Venous thromoembolism
>   Maintenance of IV catheters

Administer:
>   Adult: Blood gas syringe preparation: 0.5 ml
>   Pediatric: Check product information

Nursing Implications:
>   Assess for signs of bleeding: epitaxis, hematuria, tarry
>   stools
>   Monitor:
>   >   Activated partial thromboplastin time (PTT)
>   >   Hematocrit
>   >   Platelets
>   Protamine sulfate is antidote

Hydralazine hydrochloride

(Apresoline)
Indications in Emergencies:
>   Severe hypertension
>   Pregnancy-induced hypertension

Administer:
>   Adult: 10-40 mg IV push slowly over 4 - 5 minutes

Pediatric: 1.7 to 3.5 mg/kg/24 hours IM or IV

Nursing Implications:

Take blood pressure frequently during administration

Contraindicated with tricyclic antidepressants

Patient may experience palpitations and chest pain

Ipecac syrup

Indications in Emergenices:

Drug overdose

Poisoning

Accidental ingestion

Administer:

Adult: 30 ml PO with 1000 ml water; repeat XI.

Pediatric: 15 ml PO with 400-500 ml water; repeat X1

Infant: 10 ml PO with water; repeat X1

Nursing Implications:

If patient does not respond to repeat dose, consider gastric lavage

Check for gag reflex before administering

Do not give if ingestion is of a caustic substance, such as lye

Follow emesis with activated charcoal

Lidocaine hydrochloride

(Xylocaine)

Indications in Emergenices:

Premature ventricular contractions (PVCs)

Ventricular tachycardia

As local anesthetic agent, especially in entubation

Administer:

Adult: 25 to 100 mg IV bolus over 2 min. Can follow with 50 mg bolus 5 min later, then boluses of 50 mg every 10 min up to 325 mg; or follow first bolus with IV drip at 1-4 mg/min

Pediatric: 0.5 mg/kg over 3 min., followed by IV
 drip at 0.02 to 0.03 mg/kg/min
Nursing Implications:
 Administer via bolus following by IV drip
 Use with caution in liver disease
 Contraindicated in heart blocks
 Monitor for syncope, hypotension, bradycardia
 Use cautiously in alcoholics; treat first with thiamine

Magnesium sulfate

Indications in Emergencies:
 Pregnancy-induced hypertension (PIH)
 Hypomagnesemia
Administer:
 Adult: 4 gm IV initially, then 1-2 gm/hour
 Pediatric: Varies widely, consult product information;
  Usually not used in emergencies
Nursing Implications:
 Effects are immediate
 Monitor for hypotension, respiratory depression
 Pitocin may be ordered for inducing labor if in third
  trimester

Mannitol

(Osmitrol)
Indications in Emergencies:
 Increasing ICP
 Drug overdose
 Acute oliguric renal failure
 Intraocular pressure
Administer:
 Adult: 1.5 to 4.5 gm/kg slow IV push or 50 to 200 gm
  of 20% solution over 20 to 60 minutes

Pediatric: 2 gm/kg as a 15-20% solution over 2-6
hours, consult literature, dose will vary with
diagnosis
Nursing Implications:
Contraindicated in intracranial bleed, CHF,
pregnancy
Keep strict I & O
Monitor for hypovolemia

Meperidine hydrochloride

(Demerol)
Indications in Emergencies:
Pain relief
Administer:
Adult: 10 - 100 mg IM or IV
Nursing Implications:
Can be addictive
Give slowly IV
Monitor for hypotension, respiratory depression
Pediatric:
Not recommended

Oxytocin

(Pitocin, Syntocinon)
Indications in Emergencies:
Postpartum hemorrhage
Administer:
Adult: 10 to 20 units in D5W 100 ml (also can use
D5W and 0.45% normal saline) infusing at 0.5 to 1
ml/min.
Pediatric: Not recommended
Nursing Implications:
Watch for anaphylaxic reactions
Monitor for cardiac dysrhythmias

Can cause hypotension, tachycardia

Potassium chloride

Indications in Emergencies:
Hypokalemia
Diabetic ketoacidosis
Digitalis toxicity
Administer:
Check electrolyte balance frequently
Do not administer is renal functioning is impaired
Withhold in second-degree heart block
Withhold in dehydration or acidosis
Nursing Implications:
Watch for ventricular fibrillation, asystole
Monitor for bradycardia
May cause AV block
Decreases cell permeability

Phenytoin

(Dilantin)
Indications in Emergencies:
Status epilepticus
Cardiac dysrhythmias
Administer:
Adult: As an anticonvulsant: 150-250 mg IV over 5
min
As an antidysrhythmic: 100-300 mg IV over 24 hours
in divided doses
Pediatric: 1-2 mg/kg IV over 5 min

Quinidine gluconate

Indications in Emergencies:
Atrial flutter
Atrial fibrillation

Paroxysmal atrial tachycardia
Ventricular tachycardia
Administer:
 Adult: 800 mg in 40 ml D5W; run in 1 ml/min
 Pediatric: 30 mg/kg/24 hours in 5 divided doses
  in D5W diluted 5:1, infuse at 1 ml/min
Nursing Implications:
 Position patient supine while administering drug
 Increases prothrombin time
 Watch for adverse drug interactions, especially in conjuction with propranolol, digitalis, and procainamide

Sodium bicarbonate

Indications in Emergencies:
 Acidosis
 Cardiac arrest
 Hyperkalemia
Administer:
 Adult: Depends upon arterial pH and ventilation status
 Pediatric: Depends upon arterial pH and ventilation status
Nursing Implications:
 Do not mix with calcium chloride
 Monitor for teteny
 Causes metabolic alkalosis which is difficult to reverse

Verapamil (Isoptin)

Indications in Emergenices:
 Paroxysmal supraventricular tachycardia
Administer:
 Adult: 5 to 10 mg IV bolus slowly over 2 min; may be repeated at 0.15 mg/kg 30 min. after initial dose

Pediatric: 0.1 to 0.2 mg/kg IV slowly over 2 min; and
    consult product information for variations
Nursing Implications:
    Monitor for hypotension, bradycardia
    Watch for asystole
    Give cautionally in CHF, may worsen condition
    Do not administer in: hypotension, heart block, or
        in conjunction with beta-adrenergic drugs

DRUGS USED IN OTHER MEDICAL EMERGENCIES

Shock, hypovolemic:

Administer fluids
Consider:
Normal saline
D5LR
Blood
Albumin

Anaphylaxic shock

Epinephrine: 1:1,000 solution SC
Adults: 0.3-0.5 ml
Pediatric: 0.01 mg/kg
If shock is severe or prolonged, administer epinephrine
followed by diphenhydramine (Benadryl) 50-100 mg IM

Asthmatic attack

Epinephrine 1:1,000 solution SC
Adult: 0.3-0.5 ml q20 min x 3 doses
Pediatric: 0.01 ml/kg up to 0.30 ml/kg q 20 min x 3 doses
Bronkosol x 3 doses
or
Alupent x 3 doses

If unrelieved:
Aminophylline: Loading dose of 6 mg/kg IV for
maintenance:
Adult: 0.4-0.9 mg/kg/hr IV
Pediatric: 1.0 mg/kg/hr IV
If attack is severe or prolonged:
Hydrocortisone sodium 4 mg/kg IV q2-4h
Methylprednisolone: 2-4 mg/kg IV q4h

Narcotics overdose

Naloxone (Narcan)
Adult: 2.0 mg IV or IM; can be repeated
Pediatric: 0.01-0.02 mg/kg IV or IM

Coma of unknown cause

50 ml D5O (1 amp) IV
100 mg Thiamine

Hypertensive Crisis

Diazoxide (Hyperstat) 200-300 mg IV
Nitroprusside (Nipride) 50 mg in 500 ml, titrate drip
Hydralazine 10 mg IM
Nifedipine 10-20 mg oral or sublingual

Hypoglycemia

If patient is awake, orange juice with sugar
If no alert, 50 ml D50 (1 amp)
Treat before results of test are receive

Poisoning

Conscious:
Ipecac Syrup: Infant (1 year): 10 ml
Child (1-12- years): 15 ml
Adult: 30 ml

Lots of water
Repeat if patient does not vomit
After vomiting, activated charcoal
Child: 30 gm with 250 ml H_2O
Adult: 50 mg with 200 ml H_2O

Caution: Do not induce vomiting if poison contains
alkali, acid, petroleum or strychnine
Activated charcoal is contraindicated in Tylenol overdose

Unconscious:

Establish airway with endotracheal tube
Normal saline lavage through Ewald tube
Adults: 300 ml
Pediatric: 20 ml
Activated charcoal, if no other oral antidote is indicated
Magnesium citrate to promote GI elimination

Status Epilepticus

Diazepam (valium)
Adult: 5-10 mg IV up to 30 mg; administer: 3 mg/min
Pediatric: 0.10-0.20 IV; 1-3 mg/min

Phenytoin (Dilantin)
Adult: 15 mg IV; administer up to 50 mg/min
Pediatric: 15 mg IV watch for hypotension, bradycardia; monitor ECG

Phenobarbital
Adult: 120-140 mg IV administered at 25 mg/min
Pediatric: 10 mg IV or IM at 25 mg/min

ISOLATION PROCEDURES

Isolation techniques prevent dissemination of harmful pathogens to susceptible patients and/or health care workers by establishing barriers to these pathogens. The Centers for Disease Control issues recommendations for isolation procedures. However, hospitals will establish their own protocols for following these recommendations. Therefore, nurses may see wide variances in how the guidelines are implemented.

ASSESSMENT:

- Physician's orders and agency policy
- Medical diagnosis
- Isolation required

EQUIPMENT:

- Private room with door closed at all times
- Door sign with isolation level
- Linen gown
- Disposable gowns, masks, gloves, caps, goggles, and shoe covers
- Separate laundry hamper
- Waste container with plastic lining
- Antimicrobial soap
- Disposable, sterile utensils, dishes, tray
- Sterile linen, diagnostic tools, or any articles that will contact patient
- Isolation labels

PREPARATION:

- · Wash hands and examine for breaks in skin.
- · Identify patient.
- · Assemble equipment.
- · Explain precautions and procedures to patient, family, and visitors.
- · Place isolation sign and instructions on door.

PROCEDURES:

RATIONALE:

For infected patient:
Gown, gloves, and mask
according to isolation level.

Protects nurse from
contamination.

Elevate bed to working
level. Carry out intended
procedure or care of patient.

Provide appropriate con-
tainers for disposal of
materials.

Receives isolation materials.

Avoid vigorous movement
of bed linen.

Prevents dissemination of
pathogens by area
movement.

Dispose of all waste items,
including gloves, mask and
paper gowns before leaving
room.

Contaminated items may
not leave room until
properly disposed.

PROCEDURES:	**RATIONALE:**
With second nurse standing outside of room holding clean cuffed plastic bag, first nurse securely fastens plastic lined bag containing contaminated material. Red labels identify contents. Nurse outside room holds second bag open and first bag is dropped inside second bag.	"Double bagging" decreases possibility of contamination to environment outside of patient's room.
Remove gowns before leaving room.	Prevents transportion of pathogens.
Wash hands before untying gown ties.	Prevents spread of microorganisms.
Remove gown inside out and roll up.	Area of gown touching uniform is considered clean. By rolling, harmful pathogens are trapped inside.
For susceptible patient: Before entering room, using strict medical asepsis, wash hands.	

ISOLATION LEVELS

STRICT: Private room, gown, mask, gloves when entering, all articles in room considered contaminated. Use disposable dishes. Prevents dissemination by contact and airborne sources. Recommended most commonly in childhood diseases. Rarely used except for varicella (chickenpox), zoster (shingles), smallpox, and diphtheria.

RESPIRATORY: Private room, mask when in close contact with patient. Double bag linens and trash. All articles in room considered contaminated. Prevents dissemination by contact and airborne sources. Infections requiring respiratory isolation include measles, epiglottitis, meningitis, pneumonia, mumps, whopping cough (pertussis).

ENTERIC: Private room, gown and gloves if handling articles with feces and vomitus. Infection may spread by direct or indirect contact. Prevents dissemination by contact with contaminated articles or feces. Common infections requiring enteric isolation are amebic dysentery, cholera, diarrhea of unknown cause, encephalitis, Hepatitis A, viral meningitis and gastroenteritis.

BLOOD/BODY FLUID: Private room, gown and gloves if handling articles contaminated with blood or body fluids. Prevents dissemination by direct or indirect contact with blood or body fluids. Double bag linens and trash. Common infections requiring this isolation are AIDS, Hepatitis B and C, malaria and syphilis.

BODY SUBSTANCE: Instituted in 1987, this procedure requires masks, gloves, gowns and goggles. It is a protection against any body substance, including sweat and tears. It has largely replaced respiratory isolation.

AFB (Acid-Fast Bacilli): This is a new, highly-specialized isolation that recommends special ventilation of rooms and protective clothing. Is focuses on preventing the spread of tuberculosis. Wear gown and mask if in direct contact; gloves are not necessary. Double bag linens and trash.

DRAINAGE/SECRETION: Gown, gloves when handling drainage or secretions from any source. Prevents dissemination by contaminated articles. This procedure is not widely used because it has been incorporated into the blood/body fluid guidelines. Infections include draining wound infections such as abscesses, minor burns, decubitus ulcers and conjunctivus.

CONTACT: Private room, gown, mask, gloves for anyone in contact with patient. All articles in contact with patient are considered contaminated. Prevents dissemination by contact and airbone sources. This is the next most strict isolation. Rarely used except in mithicillin-resistant infections. Infections requiring this isolation are diphtheria, some cases of influenza, impetigo, pediculosis (lice), staph or strep pneumonia, rabies, rubella, and scabies.

NOTE: Protective or reverse isolation is not an official CDC category. However, physicians may order it on an individualized basis, especially for oncology patients.

All levels require labeling and bagging of contaminated materials.

UNIVERSAL PRECAUTIONS AGAINST AIDS

· Practice careful handwashing, before and after wearing gloves.

· Wear gloves when coming into contact with body fluids, mucous membranes, or open wounds.

· Wear gloves when handling items soiled by blood and body fluids.

· Wear gloves when skin is broken or compromised.

· Wear gloves when starting IVs and drawing blood.

- Place used needles, sharps, and scalpels in designated needle box.

- Needles are not cut and are not recapped.

- Empty needle box regularly to avoid overfilling.

- Clean up blood or body fluids with 1:10 solution of Clorox and water. This solution should be prepared daily in order to hold its strength.

- Wear masks, gowns, and goggles when involved in procedures that might produce splashes of blood or body fluids.

- Place all soiled linen in the appropriate isolation containers.

- Beware of the dangers of blood and body fluids, whether a patient has been diagnosed with AIDS or not.

HOW TO GIVE REPORT

- Keep Kardex updated.

- Always start on time.

- Use notes and / or Kardex.

- Always state:

  > Patient's name
  > Age
  > Sex
  > Room number
  > Medical diagnosis
  > Doctor's name
  > Summary of patient's chief complaint
  > Past medical history (as applicable to present problem)
  > Prioritized nursing diagnoses

- For each nursing diagnosis report significant findings:

  > Results of lab tests
  > Physical assessment
  > Treatments
  > A change in medications
  > Any scheduled diagnostic studies
  > Change in vital signs
  > Summary of discharge plan (when pertinent)

- Detail changes in patient's condition

- Briefly summarize previous nursing diagnoses that have been resolved.

- State the facts as concisely as possible, avoid judgmental descriptions.

GUIDELINES FOR QUALITY IMPROVEMENT AND CONTROL

Nursing accountability can be measured by the quality assurance process now being referred to as quality improvement. The American Nurses Association outlines a specific review process that is followed by hospitals and accrediting agencies. One of the most important agencies is the Joint Commission of Accrediting Hospital Organizations.

What is quality assurance and improvement? It is being able to measure the results of what you say you are doing. For example, if the policy and procedure states IV tubing is changed every 72 hours then the documentation should reflect that IV tubing is changed every 72 hours.

The ANA guidelines are:

- Identify values.
- Identify criteria.
- Collect data.
- Interpret data.
- Identify possible courses of action.
- Write the action plan.
- Implement the action plan.
- Reevaluate.

STANDARDS OF NURSING CARE

From the JOINT COMMISSION OF ACCREDITING HOSPITAL ORGANIZATIONS

Patients receive nursing care in various settings throughout the hospital. For example, nursing care is provided in medical-surgical nursing care units, in alcohol and other drug dependence programs, in mental health nursing care units, in biopsychosocial and physical rehabilitation programs, in hospital-sponsored ambulatory clinics and services, in emergency services, in intensive care and other special care units, and in units in which surgical and other invasive procedures are performed. The standards in this chapter apply to all settings in which nursing care is provided in the hospital.

NC.1. **PATIENTS RECEIVE NURSING CARE BASED ON A DOCUMENTED ASSESSMENT OF THEIR NEEDS.**

NC.1.1 Each patient's need for nursing care related to his/her admission is assessed by a registered nurse. The assessment is conducted either at the time of admission or within a time frame preceding or following admission that is specified in hospital policy. Aspects of data collection may be delegated by the registered nurse. Needs are reassessed when warranted by the patient's condition.

NC.1.2 Each patient's assessment includes consideration of biophysical, psychosocial, environmental, self-care, educational, and discharge planning factors. When appropriate, data from the patient's significant other(s) are included in the assessment.

NC.1.3 Each patient's nursing care is based on identified nursing diagnoses and/or patient care needs and patient care standards, and is consistent with the therapies of other disciplines. The patient and/or significant other(s) are involved in the patient's care as appropriate. Nursing staff members collaborate, as appropriate, with physicians and other clinical disciplines in making decisions regarding each patient's need for nursing care.

Throughout the patient's stay, the patient and, as appropriate, his/her significant other(s) receive education specific to the patient's health care needs. In preparation for discharge, continuing care needs are assessed and referrals for such care are documented in the patient's medical record.

The patient's medical record includes documentation of: The initial assessments and reassessments; the nursing diagnoses and/or patient care needs, the interventions identified to meet the patient's nursing care needs; the nursing care provided; the patient's response to, and the outcomes of, the care provided, and the abilities of the patient and/or, as appropriate, his/her significant other(s) to manage continuing care needs after discharge.

Nursing care data related to patient assessments, the nursing diagnoses and/or patient needs, nursing interventions, and patient outcomes are permanently integrated into the clinical information system (for example, the medical record).

Nursing care data can be identified and retrieved from the clinical information system.

NC.2 ALL MEMBERS OF THE NURSING STAFF ARE COMPETENT TO FULFILL THEIR AS-SIGNED RESPONSIBILITIES.

NC.2.1 Each member of the nursing staff is assigned clinical and/or managerial responsibilities based on educational preparation, applicable licensing laws and regulations, and an assessment of current competence.

An evaluation of each nursing staff member's competence is conducted at defined intervals throughout the individual's association with the hospital. The evaluation includes an objective assessment of the individual's performance in delivering patient care services in accordance with patient needs. The process for evaluating competence is defined in policy and procedure.

Nursing care responsibilities are assigned to a nursing staff member in accordance with:

The degree of supervision needed by the individual and its availability; and the complexity and dynamics of the condition of each patient to whom the individual is to provide services and the complexity of the assessment required by each patient, including the factors that must be considered to make appropriate decisions regarding the provision of nursing care, and the type of technology employed in providing nursing care.

NC.2.2 The determination of a nursing staff member's current clinical competence and the assignment of nursing care responsibilities are the responsibility of registered nurses who have the clinical and managerial knowledge and experience necessary to competently make these decisions.

NC.2.3 Nursing staff members participate in orientation, regularly scheduled staff meetings, and ongoing education designed to improve their competence. Participation is documented.

Appropriate nursing staff members demonstrate competence in cardiopulmonary resuscitation and other patient safety as defined by hospital policy. Competence of these nursing staff members is demonstrated and documented at least every two years. If a nursing staff member is assigned to more than one type of nursing unit or patient, the staff member is competent to provide nursing care to patients in each unit and/or to each type of patient.

Adequate and timely orientation and cross-training are provided as needed.

NC.2.4 If the hospital uses outside sources for nursing personnel, these personnel receive orientation before providing patient care.

Documented evidence of licensure and current clinical competence in assigned patient care responsibilities are reviewed and approved by the hospital before these nursing personnel engage in patient care activities. The performance of these nursing personnel in the hospital is evaluated. Responsibility for this evaluation is defined in hospital policy.

NC.3 THE NURSE EXECUTIVE AND OTHER APPROPRIATE REGISTERED NURSES DEVELOP HOSPITALWIDE PATIENT CARE PROGRAMS, POLICIES, AND PROCEDURES THAT DESCRIBE HOW THE NURSING CARE NEEDS OF PATIENTS OR PATIENT POPULATIONS ARE ASSESSED, EVALUATED, AND MET.

NC.3.1 Policies and procedures, based on nursing standards of patient care and standards of nursing practice, describe and guide the nursing care provided.

The nurse executive has the authority and responsibility for establishing standards of nursing practice. The policies, procedures, nursing standards of patient care, and standards of nursing practice are developed by the nurse executive, registered nurses, and other designated nursing staff

THE NURSE'S SURVIVAL GUIDE

members; defined in writing; approved by the nurse executive or a designee(s); used, as indicated, in the assessment of the quality of patient care; and

Review of policies and procedures include information about the relevance of policies, procedures, nursing standards of patient care, and standards of nursing practice in actual use; ethical and legal concerns; current scientific knowledge; and, findings from quality assessment and improvement activities and other evaluation mechanisms, as appropriate.

NC.3.2 Nursing staff members have a defined mechanism for addressing ethical issues in patient care. When the hospital has an ethics committee or other defined structures for addressing ethical issues in patient care, nursing staff members participate.

NC.3.3 Policies and procedures are developed in collaboration with other clinical and administrative groups, when appropriate.

The nurse executive, or a designee(s), participates in the hospital admissions system to coordinate patient requirements for nursing care with available nursing resources. In making the decision when or where to admit and/or transfer a patient, consideration is given to the ability of the nursing staff to assess and meet the patient's nursing care needs.

NC.3.4 Policies and procedures describe the mechanism used to assign nursing staff members to meet patient care needs.

There are sufficient qualified nursing staff members to meet the nursing care needs of patients throughout the hospital.

The criteria for employment, deployment, and assignment of nursing staff members are approved by the nurse executive.

Nursing staffing plans for each unit define the number and mix of nursing personnel in accordance with current patient care needs.

In designing and assessing nurse staffing plans, the hospital gives appropriate consideration to the utilization of registered nurses, licensed practical/vocational nurses, nursing assistants, and other nursing personnel, and to the potential contribution these personnel can make to the delivery of efficient and effective patient care.

The staffing schedules are reviewed and adjusted as necessary to meet defined patient needs and unusual occurrences.

Appropriate and sufficient support services are available to allow nursing staff members to meet the nursing care needs of patients and their significant other(s).

Staffing levels are adequate to support participation of nursing staff members, as assigned, in committees/meetings, and in educational and quality assessment and improvement activities.

NC.4 THE HOSPITAL'S PLAN FOR PROVIDING NURSING CARE IS DESIGNED TO SUPPORT IMPROVEMENT AND INNOVATION IN NURSING PRACTICE AND IS BASED ON BOTH THE NEEDS OF THE PATIENTS TO BE SERVED AND THE HOSPITAL'S MISSION.

NC.4.1 The plan for nurse staffing and the provision of nursing care is reviewed in detail on an annual basis and receives periodic attention as warranted by changing patient care needs and outcomes.

Registered nurses prescribe, delegate, and coordinate the nursing care provided throughout the hospital.

Consistent standards for the provision of nursing care within the hospital are used to monitor and evaluate the quality of nursing care provided throughout the hospital.

NC.4.2 The appropriateness of the hospital's plan for providing nursing care to meet patient needs is reviewed as part of the established budget review process. The review includes:

An analysis of actual staffing patterns, and findings from quality assessment and improvement activities, the allocation of financial and other resources is assessed to determine whether nursing care is provided appropriately, efficiently, and effectively, the allocation of financial and other resources is designed to support improvement and innovation in nursing practice.

NC.5 **THE NURSE EXECUTIVE AND OTHER NURSING LEADERS PARTICIPATE WITH LEADERS FROM THE GOVERNING BODY, MANAGEMENT, MEDICAL STAFF, AND CLINICAL AREAS IN THE HOSPITAL'S DECISION-MAKING STRUCTURES AND PROCESSES.**

NC.5.1 Nursing services are directed by a nurse executive who is a registered nurse qualified by advanced education and management experience.

If the hospital utilizes a decentralized organizational structure, there is an identified nurse leader at the executive level to provide authority and accountability for, and coordination of, the nurse executive functions.

When the hospital is part of a multihospital system, there is a mechanism(s) for the hospital's nurse executive to participate in policy decisions affecting patient care services at relevant levels of corporate decision making within the system.

The mechanism(s) is used to enhance the exchange of information about, as well as participation in, improving the nursing care provided to patients in the hospital. The mechanism(s) is defined in writing.

NC.5.2 The nurse executive or a designee(s) participates with leaders from the governing body, management, medical staff, and clinical areas in developing the hospital's mission, strategic plans, budgets, resource allocations, operation plans, and policies.

The nurse executive develops the nursing budget in collaboration with other nursing leaders and other hospital personnel.

The nurse executive and other nursing leaders participate in the ongoing review of the hospital's mission, strategic plans, and policies.

NC.5.3 The nurse executive and other nursing leaders participate with leaders from the governing body, management, medical staff, and clinical areas in planning, promoting, and conducting hospital wide quality monitoring and improvement activities.

Registered nurses evaluate current nursing practice and patient care delivery models to improve the quality and efficiency of patient care.

The nurse executive and other nursing leaders participate in developing and implementing mechanisms for collaboration between nursing staff members, physicians, and other clinical practitioners.

NC.5.4 The nurse executive and other nursing leaders are responsible for developing, implementing, and evaluating programs to promote the recruitment, retention, development, and continuing education of nursing staff members.

The nurse executive and other nursing leaders participate in developing and implementing mechanisms for recognizing the expertise and performance of nursing staff members engaged in patient care. The nurse executive and other nursing leaders collaborate with governing body and other management and clinical leaders to develop mechanisms for promoting the educational and advancement goals of hospital staff members.

NC.5.5 The nurse executive or a designee(s) participates in evaluating, selecting, and integrating health care technology and information management systems that support patient care needs and the efficient utilization of nursing resources.

The use of efficient interactive information management systems for nursing, other clinical (for example, dietary, pharmacy, physical therapy), and non-clinical information is facilitated wherever appropriate.

NC.5.6 When the hospital provides clinical facilities for nursing education programs, appropriate nursing leaders collaborate with nursing educators to influence curricula, including clinical and/or managerial learning experiences.

From the Accreditation Manual for Hospitals, 1992.

Used with the permission of the Joint Commission on the Accredidation of Healthcare Organizations.

NURSING

CARE PLANNING

NURSING CARE PLANNING

Table of Contents

THE NURSING PROCESS

The term "Nursing Process" was first used in 1955, and since then has become the hallmark of quality nursing care. The nursing process is a systematic, cyclic process which evolves into five steps that emphasize individualized care. Nurses are charged to the accountability of implementing the nursing process.

The five steps of the nursing process are assessment, nursing diagnosis, planning or outcome criteria, intervention, and evaluation. Each part of the process has its specific criteria for nursing action:

1. Assessing the patient's condition.
2. Identifying and stating the problem with a nursing diagnosis.
3. Planning priorities of care with specific outcome criteria.
4. Intervening to effectively implement that plan.
5. Evaluating the patient's response and outcome based upon outcome criteria.

The nursing process begins with the interview and history. When the assessment is complete, a nursing diagnosis is made, patient goals are set, outcome criteria for evaluation is determined and nursing interventions are ordered. Once this cycle is completed, reassessment is necessary. The nurse explores why and how the plan of care did or did not work.

Assessment and nursing diagnoses are the foundation of the nursing process and the nursing care plan. In order to effectively utilize nursing diagnoses, it is important to understand the three components of a nursing diagnosis, all of which must be documented. They are:

1. Statement of the problem: Identifying conditions from the NANDA list of nursing diagnoses that address independent nursing care.

2. Etiology of the problem: Identifying the probable cause of a patient's problem or potential problem.

3. Defining characteristics of the problem: Selecting the specific objective and subjective data gathered during the assessment that relate to this particular problem. Each component of the nursing process along with a specific design resulting in specific nursing actions are summarized in the following table.

THE NURSING PROCESS IN ACTION

THE PROCESS	THE DESIGN	THE ACTION
Assessment	Collect, verify and organize data. Recognize problems and potential problems. Ask the question: "What's going on with this patient in this situation?"	Interview. Patient history. Physician's history. Physical exam. Systems assessment. Lab data.

THE PROCESS	THE DESIGN	THE ACTION
Nursing Diagnosis	Specifically identify and label problems and potential problems. Ask the question: "What's the problem and the potential problem in this situation?"	Analyze data. Derive nursing diagnosis from the NANDA list. Establish the priority of problems identified.
Planning/Outcome Criteria	Plan priorities of care that are realistic for the individual. Patient-oriented goals, called outcome criteria, must be measurable and specific. These criteria are the basis upon which evaluation will be made. Ask the question: "What can the patient accomplish in this situation?"	Determine what the patient is able to achieve and ask the patient for input in the plan of care. Give the patient as much control as as possible. Delegate action and decide upon locus of decision.

THE PROCESS	THE DESIGN	THE ACTION
Intervention	What will the nurse do to help the patient accomplish care plan goals? Determine what the dependent interventions and independent interventions will be. Ask the question: "What can I do to help the patient in this situation?"	Perform nursing interventions. Begin reassessing what works and what does not. Be sure to intervene based on scientific rationales whether they are actually written on the care plan or not.
Evaluation	Determine to what extent goals have been achieved. Assess patient response. Evaluate progress based upon outcome criteria. Ask the question: "Is the patient better or worse? Why?"	Compare patient response to outcome criteria. Analyze why the patient responded the way he did. Reasssess. Update care plan. Ask the question: "What do we do now?"

THE INITIAL INTERVIEW

The purpose of the patient interview initially is to gather data, establish rapport and lay a foundation for trust between the patient and the nurse. An expression of warmth and respect by the nurse facilitates this exchange. The nurse must clearly state any expectations and assess the patient's understanding of the communication.

GUIDELINES TO THERAPEUTIC COMMUNICATION

Give the person special attention at the beginning of the intererview by calling the patient by name and using appropriate touch.

- Provide for privacy.

- Do not ask one question after another.

- Encourage the patient to talk by using silence.

- A nonjudgmental attitude is essential.

- Avoid long interviews; the patient may get tired or bored.

- Ask only one question at a time to avoid confusion.

- Avoid leading questions that suggest an expected answer.

- Avoid yes or no questions; open-ended ones are usually best.

- Use positive nonverbal communication, such as leaning forward and talking at the same eye level or maintaining eye contact without staring.

- Smile, use light humor when appropriate.

- Do not state opinions or give advice.

- Tell the patient how this information will be used.

- Actively listen to what the patient says and how he says it.

- Be aware of anxiety exhibited as nervous laughing and restlessness.

- Clarify statements when necessary, but avoid confrontation.

- Repeat important points you want the patient to remember.

- Reward the patient with positive comments at the end of the interview.

ADMISSION PATIENT HISTORY

The admission patient history needs to be taken only once and is useful when making referrals. The background information gathered will be helpful when performing the physical assessment.

BIOGRAPHICAL

Name

Age

Sex

Nationality

Significant other

Religion

Social security number

Occupation

Marital status

Referred by

Reliability of informant

Doctor's name, address

CHIEF COMPLAINT

What specific problem caused you to seek help today?

(Record as a quote exactly what the patient says)

How long has this been a problem?

DETAILED HISTORY OF ILLNESS

What: What were you doing at the time the problem occurred?

When: When did it begin (date, time of day)?

How: Was it a recurring or sudden onset? Severity?

Why: Any precipitating events that occurred?

PAST HEALTH HISTORY

Major illness (diabetes, cardiac)

Injuries in the past

Hospitalizations

Surgeries

Allergies

Immunizations

Habits: caffeine, alcohol, drugs, cigarettes

Present medications (including over-the-counter)

Nutrition/diet/weight loss or gain

Significant family illness/death

PSYCHOLOGICAL HISTORY

Cognitive:

Ability to understand

Ability to learn

Ability to remember

Coping mechanisms

Response to illness

Past coping patterns

Abusive/preventive lifestyle

SOCIOLOGICAL HISTORY

Significant relationships

Persons living at home

Recent crises/changes at home or work

Work environment: Stress/Satisfaction

Economic status

Adequate financial resources

Perception of financial needs

Financial strain of illness

Cultural/religious implications

Food preparation

Special rituals

Special religious days

COMMUNICATING WITH EMPATHY

After the initial interview, a therapeutic communication process is established. Empathetic communication is a skill acquired through self-awareness and perceptive listening. These guidelines can be integrated so the patient is the focus of the verbal and the nonverbal exchange.

GUIDELINES FOR THERAPEUTIC COMMUNICATION IN A HELPING RELATIONSHIP

- Be congruent in what you are saying and what your body language is conveying.

- Use clear, concise words that are adapted to the individual's intelligence and experience.

- Do not say, "I understand." Nonverbally or verbally say, "I care about you."

- Use appropriate silence to give the patient time to organize his thoughts.

- Let the patient set the pace of the exchange--do not hurry him.

- Accept the patient as he is. The nursing profession espouses empathy without judgment.

- Offer a collaborative relationship in which you are willing to work with the patient in resolving problems, but not for him.

- Use open-ended questions to encourage expression of feelings and thoughts.

- Explore ideas completely. Do not drop a subject that the patient has brought up without some resolution.

- Clarify statements and relationships when necessary. Do not try to read the patient's mind.

- Give positive feedback every chance you get. Praise the patient for communication and attempts at problem solving.

- Encourage expression of feelings.

- Paraphrase statements and feelings to facilitate further talking.

- Translate feelings into words so that hidden meanings can be discovered.

- Focus on reality, especially if the patient misinterprets facts or if he is misrepresenting the truth.

- Offer teaching and information, but avoid giving advice.

- Search for mutual, intuitive understanding. Encourage the patient to ask for clarification if he does not understand what is being said. Do not use phrase or slang that can be misunderstood.

- Encourage an appropriate plan of action, such as problem solving or self-care.

- Summarize at the end of the conversation to focus on the important points of the communication and validate the patient's understanding.

- Remember, the more personal and intense a feeling or thought is, the more difficult it is to communicate. Give the patient time and the security to express his deepest feelings. The key word is listen.

BARRIERS TO THERAPEUTIC COMMUNICATION

Therapeutic communication techniques are valuable. However, the attitude of caring is the foundation of therapeutic transaction. The nurse should be aware of actions that often block communication:

Using words that the patient does not understand or inappropriate cliches.

Inferring to the patient that you are in a hurry or preoccupied with other tasks.

Showing anger or anxiety, especially when these feelings provoke an argument with the patient.

Incorrectly interpreting what the patient expresses.

Offering counseling when the timing is wrong or when the patient is not ready to hear what is being communicated.

Giving false reassurance and discounting the patient's feelings.

Expressing opinions and giving advice, especially when these feelings provoke an argument with the patient.

Persistently asking probing questions that make the patient uncomfortable.

Being insincere. (Patients pick this up very quickly.)

Interrupting while the patient is talking.

DOCUMENTATION -- THE VITAL LINK TO COMMUNICATION

The purpose of charting is to communicate the care given to the patient. Documentation of nursing care must be as complete and congruent as the care itself. Documentation is the best way for a nurse to prove accountability in situations where she is responsible for patient care. The battle cry on the documentation front has become: "If it is not charted, it is not done."

WHAT TO CHART

The Head-to-Toe Systems Assessment. Get a general impression of what is going on with the patient, then focus on particular problems. Carefully assess the situation by asking yourself:

- What do I see?
- What do I hear?
- What do I think?
- What will I do?
- What should I do?
- What has already been done?
- How is the patient responding?
- The nursing process must be charted each shift by recording a nursing physical assessment, nursing diagnoses based on problems and potential problems, goals of patient care, nursing interventions and an evaluation of the patient's progress.
- Any change in condition, especially if the patient's condition is deteriorating.

- Be as specific as possible, using descriptive details rather than conveying a judgmental tone.
- Include patient response to any treatment or medication.
- Describe patient's understanding of any health teaching.
- Show continuity of care, especially with treatments that require frequent monitoring, such as IV therapy.
- Patient's medical diagnosis and treatments should be noted at least once each shift.
- Indicate all contacts with the physician, including details and direct quotes when pertinent.
- Chart exact times of patient activities, treatments or procedures.
- Chart patient care at least every two hours.
- Correlate documentation regarding the nursing care plan, physician's orders and treatment plan.

HOW TO CHART

- Always chart in the correct color of ink.
- Write legibly using accurate and concise medical terminology.
- Spell correctly.
- Addressograph and date must be on each page.
- Do not skip lines.
- Do not write between the lines.
- Do not skip times--chart in a time sequence.

- Chart at least every two hours.

- Do not chart in advance of nursing care administered.

- Close entries with name and title.

- Designate late entries as LATE ENTRY with the time.

- Make one line through an error, write ERROR, and sign.

- Never erase. Never use liquid coverup or erasable pens.

- If a page must be recopied, draw a single diagonal line across the original and designate book "copy" and "original" on the appropriate page.

- Do not chart for anyone else; never let anyone else chart for you.

- Use only those abbreviations accepted by your agency.

- Use direct quotes when appropriate.

- Be objective. Do not draw conclusions or write judgments.

- Avoid such words as "good," "normal," and "appears to be."

- The more descriptive the details, the better.

PROTECTING YOURSELF LEGALLY

There are two key elements in protecting yourself legally: documentation and respect for the patient and family. A patient who is shown respect rarely sues. However, adequate documentation is the surefire defense when a nurse is required to prove accountability.

Complete documentation will safeguard the nurse if she becomes involved in a lawsuit. The nursing notes should reflect that the nurse practiced reasonable and prudent care under the circumstances.

Biased feelings and judgmental thoughts should never be included in the nursing notes on the chart. Nurses should avoid the use of words such as "uncooperative" and "hostile." When these actions are recorded they should be written as a fact using direct quotes.

It is important that you always document that you are following the policy and procedure of the hospital. If you catherize a patient, note that it was done by sterile technique. If you change IV tubing and the policy and procedure states it should be changed every 48 hours, make a note that this was done. Every small detail of the policy and procedure does not need to be cited. However, it should be noted that a special procedure was done according to policy and procedure.

There are many reasons the nurse should know the policy and procedure of the hospital where she works. If there is a necessity for a particular policy, then it is important. Legally, it is of utmost importance to follow policy and procedure because if a nurse is involved in an incident, and she was not following policy and procedure, the hospital malpractice is not obligated to defend her. When this happens, the nurse must supply her own defense. This is one reason it is a good idea to carry private malpractice insurance.

It is essential to document any procedure that involves the patient. If it is not charted on the medical record, legally it is not done.

MORE GUIDELINES TO PREVENT MALPRACTICE

- Always exercise reasonable and prudent care under the circumstances.
- Be thoroughly knowledgeable of the hospital's policy and procedure.
- Show concern and caring about your patient.
- Show positive regard to the family. Research indicates family members are more likely to sue than the patient.
- Keep your nursing knowledge current.
- Stay knowledgeable about nursing standards of care.
- Keep current by reading nursing journals on a regular basis.
- Be selective in delegating nursing responsibilities.
- Complete charts in a timely manner.
- Always be aware of the patient's safety.
- Exercise precaution in administering medications.

NANDA APPROVED
NURSING DIAGNOSES
(TENTH CONFERENCE)

Activity intolerance

Activity intolerance: High risk for

Adjustment, impaired

Airway clearance, ineffective

Anxiety

Aspiration: High risk for

Body image disturbance

Body temperature, altered: High risk for

Breastfeeding, effective

Breastfeeding, ineffective

Breathing pattern, ineffective

Caregiver role strain

Caregiver role strain: High risk for

Communication, impaired verbal

Constipation

Constipation, colonic

Constipation, perceived

Decisional conflict (specify)

Decreased cardiac output

Defensive coping

Denial, ineffective

Diarrhea

Disuse syndrome: High risk for

Diversional activity deficit

Dysfunctional ventilatory weaning response

Dysreflexia

Family coping, compromised, ineffective

Family coping, disabling, ineffective

Family coping: Potential for growth

Family process, altered

Fatigue

Fear

Fluid volume deficit

Fluid volume deficit: High risk for

Fluid volume excess

Gas exchange, impaired

Grieving, anticipatory

Grieving, dysfunctional

Growth and development, altered

Health maintenance, altered

Health seeking behaviors (specify)

Home maintenance management, impaired

Hopelessness

Hyperthermia

Hypothermia

Inability to sustain spontaneous ventilation

Incontinence, bowel

Incontinence, functional

Incontinence, reflex

Incontinence, stress

Incontinence, total

Incontinence, urge

Individual coping, ineffective

Ineffective infant feeding pattern

Ineffective management of therapeutic regimen (individuals)

Infection: High risk for

Injury: High risk for

Injury, High risk for: Self-mutilation

Interrupted breastfeeding

Knowledge deficit (specify)

Noncompliance (specify)

Nutrition, altered: Less than body requirements

Nutrition, altered: More than body requirements

Nutrition, altered: High risk for more than body requirements

Oral mucous membrane, altered

Pain

Pain, chronic

Parental role conflict

Parenting, altered

Parenting: High risk for altered

Peripheral neurovascular dysfunction: High risk for

Personal identity disturbance

Physical mobility, impaired

Poisoning: High risk for

Posttrauma response

Powerlessness

Protection, altered

Rape-trauma syndrome

Rape-trauma syndrome: Compound reaction

Rape-trauma syndrome: Silent reaction

Relocation stress syndrome

Role performance, altered

Self-care deficit: Bathing/hygiene

Self-care deficit: Feeding

Self-care deficit: Dressing/grooming

Self-care deficit: Toileting

Self-esteem, chronic low

Self esteem, situational low

Self-esteem disturbance

Self-mutilation: High risk for

Sensory-perceptual alteration: Auditory

Sensory-perceptual alteration: Gustatory

Sensory-perceptual alteration: Kinesthetic

Sensory-perceptual alteration: Olfactory

Sensory-perceptual alteration: Tactile

Sensory-perceptual alteration: Visual

Sexual dysfunction

Sexuality patterns, altered

Skin integrity, impaired

Skin integrity, impaired: High risk for

Sleep pattern disturbance

Social interation, impaired

Social isolation

Spiritual distress (distress of the human spirit)

Suffocation: High risk for

Swallowing, impaired

Thermoregulation, ineffective

Thought processes, altered

Tissue integrity, impaired

Tissue perfusion, altered: Cardiopulmonary

Tissue perfusion, altered: Cerebral

Tissue perfusion, altered: Gastrointestinal

Tissue perfusion, altered: Peripheral

Tissue perfusion, altered: Renal

Trauma: High risk for

Unilateral neglect

Urinary elimination, altered

Urinary retention

Violence, high risk for: Self-directed or directed at others

PROFESSIONAL

NETWORK

PROFESSIONAL NETWORK

Table of Contents

HOW TO WRITE A RESUME

A resume should be concisely written and organized for at-a-glance reading. Employers quickly screen resumes, and they are often the basis for that important first impression. A professional resume consists of seven components:

I. The Cover Letter
   - Use an appropriate business letter format.
   - State the reason you are applying for the position.
   - Emphasize how your qualifications meet their requirements.
   - Request to schedule an interview.
   - State that you have enclosed your resume.

II. Personal Data
   - Name
   - Address /phone number
   - Professional license number
   - Social security number
   - Sex
   - Age
   - Race

III. Job Objectives
   - Type of position you are seeking
   - How your ability and skills qualify you for the position

IV. Educational Background
   - Where and when you went to school
   - Degrees earned

- Continuing education courses taken

V. Work Experience
- Place and dates of employment, beginning with present. Include volunteer work when applicable
- Concisely emphasize major work responsibilities

VI. Extracurricular Activities
- Personal development
- Hobbies
- Professional organizations

VII. References
- Names and addresses of three persons. Include one personal and two professional references. Avoid the names of relatives.

GUIDELINES FOR A SUCCESSFUL JOB INTERVIEW

What will the interviewer ask? The following are broad statements that will cover inqueries during the interview.

1. Tell about yourself.

    Briefly and concisely outline your strengths. Concentrate on your professional, not personal, accomplishments.

2. Tell about your qualifications for this job.

    List your strongest and most recent qualifications.

3. Tell why you want this job.

    Know something about the employer. Be able to say something positive about the company. Avoid using money as a reason.

4. Never be critical about past employers, especially if you are changing jobs. Avoid negative comments throughout the interview.

5. Tell about your ambitions. Mention that you look forward to new challenges and responsibilities.

6. Mention strengths in regards to your new position.

7. Mention weaknesses or problems that have been good experiences for you.

8. Tell about your salary expectations. Give a range based on an annual wage. De-emphasize money as your motivation for wanting the job.

BOARDS OF NURSING BY STATE

The following is a list of the state boards of nursing and continuing education requirements for each state.

STATE	BOARD OF NURSING	CE RE-QUIRE-MENTS
Alabama	Board of Nursing RSA Plaza, Suite 250 770 Washington Avenue Montgomery, AL 36130 205-242-4060	24 hours every 2 years beginning in 1993
Alaska	Board of Nursing 3601 C Street, Suite 722 Anchorage, AK 99503 907-561-2878	30 contact hours in 2 years for nurse practitioners
Arizona	Board of Nursing 2001 W. Camelback #350 Phoenix, AZ 85015 602-271-0592	None
Arkansas	State Board of Nursing 1123 South University Suite 800 Little Rock, AR 72204 501-686-2700	None
California	Board of Nursing Box 944210 Sacramento, CA 94244-2100 916-322-3350	30 contact hours every two years
Colorado	Board of Nursing 1560 Broadway Suite 670 Denver, CO 80202 303-894-2430	20 contact hours every 2 years

Connecticut	Board of Nursing 150 Washington Hartford, CT 06106 203-566-1041	None
Delaware	Board of Nursing Margaret O'Neil Building Box 1401 Dover, DE 19903 302-739-4522	30 contact hours every 2 years
District of Columbia	Nurses Examining Board 614 H Street, N.W. Rm. 112 Washington, D.C. 20001 202-727-7823	None
Florida	Board of Nursing 111 East Coastline Drive Suite 516 Jacksonville, FL 32202 904-359-6341	24 contact hours every 2 years
Georgia	Board of Nursing 166 Pryor Street, S.W. Suite 400 Atlanta, GA 30303 404-656-3943	None
Hawaii	Board of Nursing Box 3469 Honolulu, HI 96801 808-548-7471	None
Idaho	Board of Nursing 280 North 8th Street, Suite 210 Boise, ID 83720 208-334-3110	Nurse prac- titioners 60 contact hours every 2 years

Illinois	Department of Professional Regulation 320 West Washington Street Third Floor Springfield, IL 62786 217-782-0458	None
Indiana	Board of Nurses Registration One American Square, Suite 1020 Indianapolis, IN 46282 317-232-2960	None
Iowa	Board of Nursing 1223 E. Court Avenue Des Moines, IA 50319 515-281-3255	45 contact hours every 3 years
Kansas	Board of Nursing P.O. Box 1098 503 Kansas Avenue, Suite 330 Topeka, KS 66601 913-296-4929	30 contact hours every 2 years
Kentucky	Board of Nursing 4010 DuPont Circle, Suite 430 Louisville, KY 40207 502-897-5143	30 contact hours every 2 years, including 2 hours of HIV/AIDS education
Louisiana	Board of Nursing 150 Baronne Street, Room 912 New Orleans, LA 70112 504-568-5464	30 contact years every 2 years, or 20 hours plus 320 hours active practice

Maine	Board of Nursing 158 State House Station Augusta, ME 04333 207-289-5324	None
Maryland	Board of Nursing 201 West Preston Street Baltimore, MD 21201 301-383-2084	None
Massachus- setts	Board of Registration in Nursing Leverett Saltonstall Bldg., Government Center 100 Cambridge Street Boston, MA 02202 617-727-9961	15 contact hours every 2 years
Michigan	Board of Nursing Box 30018 905 Southland Lansing, MI 48909 517-373-1600	None
Minnesota	Board of Nursing 2700 University Ave. West #108 St. Paul, MN 55114 612-642-0575	30 contact hours every 2 years
Mississippi	Board of Nursing 239 N. Lamar Number 401 Jackson, MS 39201 601-359-6170	Nurse prac- titioners 40 hours every 2 years
Missouri	Board of Nursing Box 656 3523 N. Ten Mile Drive Jefferson City, MO 65102 314-751-0681	None

Montana	Board of Nursing 111 North Jackson Arcade Building, Lower Level Helena, MT 59620 406-444-2071	None
New York		
Nebraska	Department of Health Bureau of Examining Boards 301 Centennial Mall P.O. Box 95007 Lincoln, NE 68509 402-471-2115	20 contact hours and 200 hours of nurs- ing practice every 5 years, or 75 contact hours
Nevada	Board of Nursing 1281 Terminal Way Suite 116 Reno, NV 89502 702-786-2778	30 contact hours every 2 years
New Hampshire	Board of Nursing Education and Registration 105 Loudon Road Concord, NH 03301 603-271-2323	Nurse prac- titioners 20 hours every 2 years
New Jersey	Board of Nursing 1100 Raymond Blvd., Room 319 Newark, NJ 07102 201-648-2490	None
New Mexico	Board of Nursing 4523 Montgomery NE Suite 130 Albuquerque, NM 87109 505-841-8340	30 hours every 2 years; 50 hours for nurse practitioners

New York	Board for Nursing State Education Department Cultural Education Center Albany, NY 12230 518-474-3848	None
North Carolina	Board of Nursing P.O. Box 2129 Raleigh, NC 27602 919-782-3211	None
North Dakota	Board of Nursing 418 East Rosser Avenue Bismark, ND 58505 701-224-2974	None
Ohio	Board of Nursing Education and Registration 65 South Front Street, Suite 509 Columbus, OH 43215 614-466-3947	None
Oklahoma	Board of Nursing 2915 North Classen, Suite 524 Oklahoma City, OK 73106 405-525-2076	None
Oregon	Board of Nursing 10445 S.W. Canyon Road Beaverton, OR 97005 503-644-2767	Nurse prac- titioners 100 contact hours every 2 years
Pennsylvania	State Board of Nursing P.O. Box 2649 Harrisburg, PA 17105-2649 717-783-7142	None

Rhode Island	Board of Nursing Professional Regulation 3 Capitol Hill, Room 104 Providence RI 02908 401-277-2827	None
South Carolina	Board of Nursing 220 Executive Center Drive Columbia, SC 29210-8420 803-731-1648	None
South Dakota	Board of Nursing 3307 South Lincoln Sioux Falls, SD 57105-5224 605-335-4973 Fax 605-335-2977	None
Tennessee	Board of Nursing 283 Plus Park Blvd. Nashville, TN 37129-5407 615-367-6232	None
Texas	Board of Nurse Examiners 1901 Burnet Road, Suite 104 Austin, TX 78758 or (mailing address) Box 140466 Austin, TX 78714 512-835-4880	20 contact hours every 2 years
Utah	Department of Commerce Division of Occupational and Professional Licensing 160 East 300 South Salt Lake City, UT 84145- 0805 801-530-6628	Must work 1200 hours

Vermont	Board of Nursing 109 State Street Montpelier, VT 05609-1106 In Vermont: 800-439-8683 Outside: 802-828-2396	CEU: None Practice require- ment: 400 hours in 2 years or 960 hours in 5 years
Virginia	Board of Nursing 1601 Rolling Hills Drive Richmond, VA 23229 804-662-9909	None
Washington	Board of Nursing Box 1099 Olympia, WA 98507-1099 206-753-3726	None
West Virginia	Board of Examiners Embleton Building, Room 309 922 Quarrier Street Charleston, WV 25301 304-348-3596	None
Wisconsin	Department of Regulation and Licensing Board of Nursing P.O. Box 8935 Madison, WI 53708 608-266-0257	None
Wyoming	State Board of Nursing 2301 Central Avenue Barrett Building, 2nd Floor Cheyenne, WY 82002-0054 307-777-7601	20 hours in 2 years or prac- tice for 500 hrs. in 2 years or 1600 hrs. in 5 yrs or pass RNNCLEX within last 5 yrs.

STATE NURSES ASSOCIATIONS

The American Nurses Association is supported by the following 53 state organizations.

Alabama State Nurses Assn.
360 North Hull Street
Montgomery, Alabama 36197
(205) 262-8321

Alaska Nurses Assn.
237 East Third Avenue
Anchorage, Alaska 99501
(907) 274-0827

Arizona Nurses Assn.
1850 E. Southern Ave., Suite 1
Tempe, Arizona 85282
(602) 831-0404

Arkansas State Nurses Assn.
117 South Cedar Street
Little Rock, Arkansas 72205
(501) 664-5853

California Nurses Assn.
1855 Folsom Street, Suite 670
San Francisco, California 94103
(415) 864-4141

Colorado Nurses Assn.
5453 East Evans Place
Denver, Colorado 80222
(303) 757-7484

Connecticut Nurses Assn.
Meritech Business Park
377 Research Pkwy, Suite 2D
Meriden, Connecticut 06450
(203) 238-1207

Delaware Nurses Assn.
2634 Capitol Trail, Suite A
Newark, Delaware 19711
(302) 368-2333

District of Columbia Nurses
Assn.
5100 Wisconsin Ave. NW,
Suite 306
Washington, D.C. 20016
(202) 244-2705

Florida Nurses Assn.
P.O. Box 536985
Orlando, Florida 32853-6985
(305) 896-3261

Georgia Nurses Assn.
1362 West Peachtree Street, N.W.
Atlanta, Georgia 30309
(404) 876-4624

Guam Nurses Assn.
P.O. Box 3134
Agana, Guam 96910

Hawaii Nurses Assn.
677 Ala Moana Blvd., Suite 301
Honolulu, Hawaii 96813
(808) 531-1628 or 521-8361

Idaho Nurses Assn.
200 North 4th St., Suite 20
Boise, Idaho 83702-6001
(208) 345-0500

Illinois Nurses Assn.
20 North Wacker Drive,
Suite 2520
Chicago, Illinois 60606
(312) 236-9708

Indiana State Nurses Assn.
2915 North High School Road
Indianapolis, Indiana 46224
(317) 299-4575

Iowa Nurses Assn.
100 Court Avenue, 9LL
Des Moines, Iowa   50309
(515) 282-9169

Kansas State Nurses Assn.
700 S.W. Jackson, Suite 601
Topeka, Kansas 66603
(913) 233-8638

Kentucky Nurses Assn.
1400 South First Street
Louisville, Kentucky   40201
(502) 637-2546

Louisiana State Nurses Assn.
712 Transcontinental Drive
Metairie, Louisiana 70001
(504) 889-1030

Maine State Nurses Assn.
P.O. Box 2240
Augusta, Maine 04330
(207) 622-1057

Maryland Nurses Assn.
5820 Southwestern Boulevard
Baltimore, Maryland 21227
(301) 242-7300

Massachusetts Nurses Assn.
340 Turnpike Street
Canton, Massachusetts 02021
(617) 821-4625

Michigan Nurses Assn.
120 Spartan Avenue
East Lansing, Michigan 48823

Minnesota Nurses Assn.
1295 Bandana Blvd. North,
Suite 140
St. Paul, Minnesota 55108-5115
(612) 646-4807

Mississippi Nurses Assn.
135 Bounds Street, Suite 100
Jackson, Mississippi 39206
(601) 982-9182

Missouri Nurses Assn.
206 East Dunklin St. Box 325
Jefferson City, Missouri 65101
(314) 636-4623

Montana Nurses Assn.
104 Broadway, Suite G-2
P.O. Box 5718
Helena, Montana 59601
(406) 442-6710

Nebraska Nurses Assn.
941 "O" Street, Suite 707-711
Lincoln, Nebraska 68508
(402) 475-3859

Nevada Nurses Assn.
3660 Baker Lane, Suite 104
Reno, Nevada 89509
(702) 825-3555

New Hampshire Nurses Assn.
48 West Street
Concord, New Hampshire 03301
(603) 225-3783

New Jersey State Nurses Assn.
320 West State Street
Trenton, New Jersey, 87108
(505) 268-7744

New Mexico Nurses Assn.
303 Washington S.E.
Albuquerque, New Mexico 87108

New York State Nurses Assn.
2113 Western Avenue
Guilderland, New York 12084
(518) 456-5371

North Carolina Nurses Assn.
Box 12025
103 Enterprise Street
Raleigh, North Carolina 27605
(919) 821-4250

North Dakota State Nurses Assn.
Green Tree Square
212 North Fourth Street
Bismarck, North Dakota 58501
(701) 223-1385

Ohio Nurses Assn.
4000 East Main Street
Columbus, Ohio 43213-2950
(614) 237-5414

Oklahoma Nurses Assn.
6414 North Santa Fe., Suite A
Oklahoma City, Oklahoma 73116
(405) 840-3476

Oregon Nurses Assn.
9600 S.W. Oak, Suite 550
Portland, Oregon 97223
(503) 293-0011

Pennsylvania Nurses Assn.
2578 Interstate Drive
P.O. Box 8525
Harrisburg, Pennsylvania 17105-
8525
(717) 657-1222

Rhode Island State Nurses Assn.
Hall Building South
354 Blackstone Boulevard
Providence, Rhode Island 02906
(401) 421-9703

South Carolina Nurses Assn.
1821 Gadsden Street
Columbia, South Carolina 29201

South Dakota Nurses Assn.
1505 South Minnesota, Suite #6
Sioux Falls, South Dakota 57105
(605) 338-1401

Tennessee Nurses Assn.
545 Mainstream Drive, Suite 405
Nashville, Tennessee 37228-1207
(615) 254-0350

Texas Nurses Assn.
Community Bank Building
300 Highland Mall Blvd.,
Suite 300
Austin, Texas 78752-3718
(512) 452-0645

Utah Nurses Assn.
1058A East 900 South
Salt Lake City, Utah 84105
(801) 322-3439

Vermont State Nurses Assn.
500 Dorset Street
South Burlington, Vermont
05403
(802) 864-9390

Virgin Islands Nurses Assn.
P.O. Box 583
Christiansted
St. Croix, U.S. VI 00820
(809) 773-2323 ext. 154
Virginia Nurses Assn.
1311 High Point Avenue
Richmond, Virginia 23230
(804) 353-7311

Washington State Nurses Assn.
2505 Second Avenue, Suite 500
Seattle, Washington 98121
(206) 443-9762

West Virgina Nurses Assn.
1 Players Club Drive, Bldg. #3
P.O. Box 1946
Charleston, West Virginia 25327
(304) 342-1169

Wisconsin Nurses Assn.
6117 Monona Drive
Madison, Wisconsin 53716
(608) 221-0383

Wyoming Nurses Assn.
Majestic Building, Room 305
1603 Capitol Avenue
Cheyenne, Wyoming 82001
(307) 635-3955

Virgin Islands Nurses Assn.
P.O. Box 2866
Charlotte Amalie
St. Thomas, Virgin Islands 00801

*SOURCE: THE AMERICAN NURSES ASSOCIATION, 1992

NURSING ORGANIZATIONS

Aerospace Medical Assn.
Flight Nurse Section
Washington National Airport
Washington, DC   20001

Alpha Tau Delta
National Fraternity for Professional Nurses
489 Serento Circle
Thousand Oaks, CA 91360

American Assn. of Colleges of Nursing
Suite 430
11 DuPont Circle
Washington, DC 20036

American Assn. of Critical Care Nurses
One Civic Plaza
New Port Beach, CA   92660

American Assn. of Nephrology Nurses
Box 56
N Woodbury Road
Pitman, NJ 08071

American Assn. of Neurological/Neurosurgical Nurses
Suite 1519
625 N. Michigan Ave.
Chicago, IL 60611

American Assn. of Nurse Anesthetists
Suite 929
111 E. Wacker Drive
Chicago, IL. 60601

American College of Nurse Midwives
Suite 1120
1522 K Street NW
Washington, DC 20005

American Holistic Nurses Assn.
P.O. Box 116
Telluride, CO 81435

American Indian Nurses Assn.
P.O. Box 1588
Norman, OK 73071

American Nurses Association, Inc.
1101 N. 14th St. NW, Suite 700
Washington, DC 20005

American Society for Nursing
Service Administrators
840 N Lakeshore Drive
Chicago, IL 60611

Association for Practitioners in Infection Control
23341 N Milwaukee Avenue
Half Day, IL 60069

Association of Operating Room Nurses
10170 E Mississippi Avenue
Denver, CO 80231

Association of Pediatric Oncology Nurses
P.O. Box 7999
San Francisco, CA 94120

Association of Rehabilitation Nurses
Suite 470
1701 Lake Avenue
Glenview, IL 60025

National Organization for the Advancement
of Associate Degree Nursing (NOAADN)
Amarillo College
P.O. Box 447
Amarillo, TX 79178

Emergency Department Nurses Assn.
Suite 1131
666 N. Lakeshore Dr.
Chicago, IL 60611

International Assn. for Enterostomal Therapy
1701 Lake Avenue
Glenview, IL 60025

International Council of Nurses
3, rue Ancien-Port 1201
Geneva, Switzerland

North American Nursing Diagnosis Assn.
St. Louis University
Dept. of Nursing
3525 Caroline St.
St Louis, MO 63104

North Assn. of Hispanic Nurses
4359 S. Rockdale
San Antonio, TX 78233

National Assn. of Pediatric Nurses Associates/Practitioners
Box 56
N Woodbury Road
Pitman, NJ 08071

National Black Nurses Assn.
425 Ohio Building
175 South Main Street
Akron, OH 44308

National Center for Nursing Ethics
PO Box 2237
Cincinnati, OH 45201

National League for Nursing
10 Columbus Circle
New York, NY 10019

National Male Nurses Assn.
2308 State Street
Saginaw, MI 48502

National Nurses Society on Alcoholism
PO Box 7728
Indian Branch Creek
Shawnee Mission, KS 66207

National Student Nurses Assn.
Suite 1325
555 W. 57th St.
New York, NY 10019

Nurses Christian Fellowship
233 Langdon St.
Madison, WI 53703

Oncology Nursing Society
701 Washington Road
Pittsburgh, Pa. 15228

Orthopedic Nurses Assn.
Suite 501
1938 Peach Tree Road NW
Atlanta, GA   30309

Sigma Theta Tau
National Honor Society of Nursing
P.O. Box 1926
Indianapolis, IN   46206-1926

World Health Organization
Avenue Appia 1211
Geneva 27, Switzerland

National Licensed Practical Nurses Educational Foundation
888 7th Avenue
New York, NY   10019

CLINICAL REFERRALS

Clinical Referrals

Table of Contents

MEDICAL HOTLINES

Organization	Hotline Number	Services Offered
AIDS Hotline	800-324-2437	Educational materials, crisis intervention counseling
Alzheimer's	800-272-3900	Emotional support, referrals to support services
American Council on Alcoholism	800-527-5344	Answers questions, referral system
American Diabetes Assn.	800-232-3472	Answers questions, provides a wide variety of patient education tools
Juvenile Diabetes Assn.	800-223-1138 in New York: 212-889-7575	Provides referrals and wide variety of educational materials
Arthritis Medical Center	800-327-3027	Answers questions, provides patient education, some referrals

Organization	Hotline Number	Services Offered
American Kidney Fund	800-638-8299	Information, financial assistance to dialysis patients
American Liver Foundation	800-223-0179	Information, physician referrals, raises funds for research
Bulemia-Anorexia Self-Help (BASH)	800-227-4785	Information, referrals
Cancer Information Service	(800) 422-6237	Answers questions, education material, support services
Compassionate Friends	708-990-0010	Referral to support groups for parents whose children have died
Depressive Illness Foundation, Inc.	800-248-4344	Educational materials
Down's Syndrome	800-221-4602	Organizes support groups; provides information
Dyslexia Society	800-222-3123	Information, referral system

Organization	Hotline Number	Services Offered
Epilepsy Foundation of America	800-332-1000	Educational material for teachers and nurses, discount pharmacy services
Hearing and Speech Action	800-638-8255	Organizes support groups and patient education, Some referrals
Hill-Burton Free Hospital Care	800-638-0742	Helps to pay hospital bills, hears Medicare complaints
Lung Hotline (National Jewish Hospital/Asthma Center)	800-222-5864	Answers questions about respiratory and immune system
Lupus Foundation of America	800-558-0121	Information
Medicare Hotline (Health Care Financing Administration)	800-638-6833	Provides system of referrals, especially for second opinions
Missing, Exploited Children	800-843-5678	Information, case management

Organization	Hotline Number	Services Offered
National Child Safety Council	800-327-5107	Distribution of educational material through local law enforcement officials
National Council of Compulsive Gambling	800-522-4700	Information, list of treatment center, therapists, referral to support groups
National Health Information	(800) 336-4797	Provides patient education materials, answers questions, offers referrals
National Institute on Drug Abuse	800-662-4357	Educational materials, some referrals
National Multiple Sclerosis Society	800-227-3166	Information, support system
National Parkinson Foundation	800-327-4545	Information, physician referral, physician support group referral
National Reyes Syndrome Foundation	800-233-7393	Educational material

Organization	Hotline Number	Services Offered
National Sexually Transmitted Disease	800-227-8922	Answers questions, educational material
National Sudden Infant Death Syndrome Foundation	800-221-7437	Family, support services, referrals for grief counseling, research, crisis intervention
National Spinal Cord Injury	800-526-3456	Referral system, peer support groups
Organ Donor	800-243-6667	Donor cards, educational material for patients
Poison Hotline (National Poison Center Network)	800-962-1253 also: 412-681-6669	Answers questions, offers referrals
Parent's Anonymous	800-421-0353	Referral to support groups
SHARE	314-947-5000	Pregnancy and infant loss support groups
Spina Bifida Assn.	800-621-3141	Educational materials, patient newsletter

Organization	Hotline Number	Services Offered
U.S. Public Health Service	800-336-4797	Recorded messages, referrals
Vietnam Veterans of America	800-424-7275	Information, crisis intervention, referrals to local support groups

ORGANIZATIONS FOR
SPECIFIC DISEASES

The following is a list of addresses of organizations devoted to patient education of specific diseases.

Alcoholism   Al-Anon, Family Group Headquarters
                              1 Park Avenue
                              New York, New York 10016
                              (800) 356-9996

                              Alcoholics Anonymous
                              15 E. 26 St. #1828
                              New York, New York 10017
                              (212) 683-3900

                              National Council on Alcoholism
                              12 W. 21st St.
                              New York, New York 10010
                              (212) 206-6770

ALLERGY   Asthma and Allergy Foundation of
                              America
                              9604 Wisconsin Avenue
                              Bethesda, Maryland 20205

ALZHEIMER'S DIS-   Alzheimer's Disease and Related
EASE   Disorders Association
                              551 Fifth Avenue
                              New York, New York 10176
                              (212) 983-0700

ARTHRITIS   Arthritis Foundation
                              3400 Peachtree Road, N.E.
                              Atlanta, Georgia 30326

ASTHMA	National Asthma Center 3800 E. Colfax Avenue Denver, Colorado 80206 (303) 388-4461
	National Foundation for Asthma P.O. Box 50304 Tucson, Arizona 85703
AUTISM	National Society for Autistic Childern Suite 1017 1234 Massachusetts Avenue, N.W. Washington, D.C. 20005
BIRTH DEFECTS	National Foundation March of Dimes Box 200 White Plains, New York 10602
	National Genetics Foundation, Inc. 250 West 57th Street New York, New York 10019
BLINDNESS	American Foundation for the Blind 15 West 16th Street New York, New York 10011 (212) 620-2000
	National Society for the Prevention of Blindness 79 Madison Avenue New York, New York 10016
BLOOD	American Association of Blood Banks 1117 N. 19th Street Suite 600 Arlington, Virginia 22209 (703) 528-8200
	Blood Research Foundation 1750 Pennsylvania Avenue, N.W. Washington, D.C. 20006

BRAIN DISEASE- MINIMAL BRAIN DYSFUNCTION	Association for Children With Learning Dysfunction 4156 Library Road Pittsburgh, Pennsylvania 15234 (412) 341-1515
	National Easter Seal Society 23 West Ogden Avenue Chicago, Illinois 60612 (312) 243-8400
BURNS	American Burn Association New York Hospital-Cornell Medical Center 525 East 68th Street, Rm. F758 New York, New York 10021 (212) 744-4447
	International Society for Burn Injuries 4200 East Ninth Avenue, C309 Denver, Colorado 80262
CANCER	American Association for Cancer Education, Inc. Albany Medical College Albany, New York 12208 (518) 445-3188
	American Cancer Society 777 Third Avenue New York, New York 10017
	Candlelighters Foundation 1312 18th St. N.W., Suite 200 Washington, DC 20036 (202) 659-5136
	Leukemia Society of America, Inc. 800 Second Avenue New York, New York 10017

Ronald McDonald House
500 North Michigan Avenue
Chicago, Illinois 60611
(312) 836-7100

CEREBRAL PALSY   United Cerebral Palsy Association
66 East 34th Street
New York, New York 10016

United Cerebral Palsy Association
The National Easter Seal Society For
Crippled Children and Adults
2023 Ogden Avenue
Chicago, Illinois 60612
(312) 243-8400

CLEFT PALATE   American Cleft Palate Association
1218 Grandview Avenue
University of Pittsburgh
Pittsburgh, Pennsylvania 15211
(412) 481-1376

CYSTIC FIBROSIS   National Cystic Fibrosis Foundation
Suite 309
6000 Executive Boulevard
Rockville, Maryland 20852

Cystic Fibrosis Foundation
60 East 42nd Street, Room 1563
New York, New York 10165
(212) 986-8783

DEAFNESS   Alexander Graham Bell Association
for the Deaf, Inc.
3417 Volta Place, NW
Washington, DC 20007
(202) 337-5220

American Deafness and Rehabilitation
Association
814 Thayer Avenue
Silver Spring, Maryland 20910
(501) 663-4617

DIABETES

American Diabetes Association
505 8th Avenue
New York, New York 10018
(212) 947-9707

Juvenile Diabetes Foundation
432 Park Avenue
New York, New York 10010
(212) 889-7575

DOWN'S SYNDROME

National Association for
Down's Syndrome
P.O. Box 63
Oak Park, Illinois 60303
(312) 543-6060

ELDERLY

Grey Panthers
3635 Chestnut Street
Philadelphia, Pennsylvania 19104

National Council on the Aging
600 Maryland Avenue, S.W.
Washington, D.C. 20024
(202) 479-1200

EMPHYSEMA

Emphysema Anonymous
1364 Palmetto Avenue
Ft. Myers, Florida 33902

EPILEPSY

American Epilepsy Society
Dept. of Neurology
Reed Neurological Research Center
710 Westwood Plaza
Los Angeles, California 90024
(213) 825-5745

Epilepsy Foundation of American
Suite 406
4351 Garden City Drive
Landover, Maryland 20785
(301) 459-3700

HEADACHE

National Migraine Foundation
5252 North Western Avenue
Chicago, Illinois 60625
(312) 878-7715

HEAD INJURY

National Head Injury Foundation
280 Singletary Lane
Framingham, Massachusetts 01701

HEART DISEASE

American Heart Association
7320 Greenville Avenue
Dallas, Texas 75231
(214) 373-6300

Mended Hearts
721 Huntington Avenue
Boston, Massachusetts 02115
(617) 732-5609

HEMOPHILIA

National Hemophilia Foundation
19 West 34th Street
New York, New York 10001

HUNTINGTON'S DISEASE	Hereditary Disease Foundation Suite 1204 9701 Wilshire Boulevard Beverly Hills, California 90212
	National Huntington's Disease Association 128 A East 74th Street New York, New York 10021
KIDNEY	National Association of Patients on Hemodialysis and Transplantation 505 Northern Boulevard Great Neck, New York 11021
	National Kidney Foundation 30 E. 33rd Street New York, New York 10016 (212) 889-2210
LIVER	American Association for the Study of Liver Disease Veterans Administration Hospital First Avenue at East 24th Street New York, New York 10010
	The Children's Liver Foundation 28 Highland Avenue Maplewood, New Jersey 07040 (800) 526-1593
LUNG	American Lung Association 1740 Broadway New York, New York 10019 (212) 315-8700

Black Lung Association
2 Hale Street
Charleston, West Virgina 25301
(304) 347-7100

LUPUS

National Lupus Erythematosus
Foundation
Suite 206
5430 Van Nuys Boulevard
Van Nuys, California 91401

National Lupus Foundation
P.O. Box 2058
Falls Church, Virginia 22042

MATERNAL AND
CHILD HEALTH

American Association for
Maternal and Child Health, Inc.
P.O. Box 965
Los Altos, California 94022
(415) 964-4575

Association for Children with
Learning Disabilities
4156 Library Road
Pittsburgh, Pennsylvania 15234
(412) 341-1515

LeLeche League International
9616 Minneapolis Avenue
Franklin Park, Illinois 60131
(312) 455-7730

MENTAL HEALTH

Recovery, Inc. (Association of
Nervous and Former Mental Patients)
116 South Michigan Avenue
Chicago, Illinois 60603

MULTIPLE SCLEROSIS	National Multiple Sclerosis Society 733 3rd Avenue New York, New York 10017 (212) 986-3240
MUSCULAR DYSTROPHY	Muscular Dystrophy Association Incorporated 3561 E. Sunrise Drive Tucson, Arizona 85718 (602) 529-2000
MYASTHENIA GRAVIS	Myasthenia Gravis Foundation Incorporated 15 East 26th Street New York, New York 10010
NARCOLEPSY	American Narcolepsy Association 425 California Street, Suite 201 San Francisco, California 94104 (415) 591-7979
NUTRITION	American Dietetic Association 430 North Michigan Avenue Chicago, Illinois 60611 (312) 899-0040
PARAPLEGIA	National Spinal Cord Injury Foundation 369 Elliot Street Newton Upper Falls, Massachusetts 02164 (671) 935-2722
PARKINSON'S DISEASE	American Parkinson's Disease Suite 417 116 John Street New York, New York 10038 (718) 981-8001

National Parkinson Foundation
1501 N.W. Ninth Avenue
Miami, Florida 33136
(305) 547-6666

PEPTIC ULCER

Center for Ulcer Research and Educa-
tion
Building 115, Room 1117 B
VA Wadsworth Hospital
Los Angeles, California 90074
(213) 825-5091

National Institute of Arthritis,
Diabetes, and Digestive and Kidney
Diseases
National Institutes of Health
Bethesda, Maryland 20205
(301) 496-4000

PHOBIAS

The Phobias Clinic
White Plains Hospital
Davis Avenue & East Post Road
White Plains, New York 10601
(914) 681-1038

PSORIASIS

National Psoriasis Foundation
Suite 210
6443 S.W. Beaverton Hwy.
Portland, Oregon 97221
(503) 297-1545

Psoriasis Research Foundation
107 Vista del Grande
San Carlos, California 94070
(415) 593-1394

RESPIRATORY DISEASES	American Association for Respiratory Therapy 11030 Ables Lane Dallas, Texas 75229 (214) 315-8700
	American Lung Association 1740 Broadway New York, New York 10019 (212) 245-8000
REYE'S SYNDROME	American Reye's Syndrome Assn. Suite 203 701 South Logan Denver, Colorado 80209
	National Reye's Syndrome Foundation 426 N. Lewis Bryan, Ohio 43506 (419) 636-2679
SCHIZOPHRENIA	Schizophrenia Foundation of New York 105 East 22nd Street New York, New York
SICKLE CELL ANEMIA	The Sickle Cell Disease Foundation of Greater New York 127 W. 127th St. New York, New York 10027 (212) 865-1500
SPINA BIFIDA	Spina Bifida Association of America Suite 317 343 South Dearborn Chicago, IL 60604

SPINAL CORD   National Spinal Cord Injury Founda-
INJURY   tion
                       600 W. Cummin, Suite 200
                       Wolburn, Massachussetts 01801
                       (617) 935-2722

STROKE   American Heart Association
                       7320 Greenville Avenue
                       Dallas, Texas 75231
                       (214) 750-5300

                       The Stroke Foundation, Incorporated
                       898 Park Avenue
                       New York, New York 10021
                       (212) 734-3461

SUDDEN INFANT   National Sudden Infant Death
DEATH SYNDROME   Syndrome Foundation
                       310 South Michigan Avenue
                       Chicago, Illinois 60604
                       (312) 663-0650

TAY-SACHS   National Tay-Sachs and Allied
                       Diseases Association, Inc.
                       122 East 42nd Street
                       New York, New York 10168
                       (212) 661-2780

VENEREAL DISEASES   American Social Health Assn.
                       260 Sheridan Avenue
                       Palo Alto, California 94306
                       (415) 321-5134

FEDERAL HEALTH AGENCIES

The following list of federal offices handle health-related problems and are a useful resource of information. When contacting these offices, ask for the Information Officer.

Alcohol, Drug Abuse and Mental
Health Administration
Parklawn Building
5600 Fishers Lane
Rockville, Maryland 20857
(301) 443-2403

National Institute on
Mental Health
17-105 Parklawn Building
5600 Fishers Lane
Rockville, Maryland 20857
(301) 443-3673

National Institute on Alcohol
Abuse And Alcoholism
16-05 Parklawn Building
5600 Fishers Lane
Rockville, Maryland 20857
(301) 443-3885

National Institute on Drug Abuse
10-05 Parklawn Buiding
5600 Fishers Lane
Rockville, Maryland 20857
(301) 443-6480

Centers for Disease Control
2000 Building 1
1600 Clifton Road, NE
Atlanta, Georgia 30333
(404) 639-3311

Food and Drug Administration
Parklawn Building
5600 Fishers Lane
Rockville, Maryland 20857
(301) 443-2404

Bureau of Drugs
138-45 Parklawn Building
5600 Fishers Lane
Rockville, Maryland 20857
(301) 443-2894

Health Services Administration
Parklawn Building
5600 Fishers Lane
Rockville, Maryland 20857
(301) 443-2065

Bureau of Community
Health Services
7-05 Parklawn Building
5600 Fishers Lane
Rockville, Maryland 20857
(301) 443-320

Health Care Financing Administration
314G Hubert H. Humphrey Building
200 Independence Avenue, SW
Washington, D.C. 20201
(202) 245-6726

Health Resources Administration
Center Building
700 East-West Hwy.
Hyattsville, Maryland 20872
(301) 436-8988

National Institutes of Health
9000 Rockville Pike
Bethesda, Maryland 20892
(301) 496-4000

National Library of Medicine Office of Inquiries and
Publications Management
M121 Building 38
8600 Rockville Pike
Bethesda, Maryland 20894
(301) 496-6308

OSHA
Occupational Safety and Health Administration
Dept of Labor
200 Constitution Ave. NW
N-36-47
Washington, D.C. 20010
(202) 523-8148

NURSING JOURNALS

The following is a list of the most prominent nursing journals available.

AMERICAN NURSE
American Nurses Assn.
1101 14th Street N.W., Suite 700
Washington, DC   20005

AMERICAN JOURNAL OF NURSING
P.O. Box 1726
Riverton, NJ   08077-7326

ARCHIVES OF PSYCHIATRIC NURSING
Editorial:
W.B. Saunders Co.
The Curtis Center
Independence Square West
Philadelphia, PA   19106-3399

Subscriptions:
W.B. Saunders Co.
6277 Sea Harbor Dr.
Orlando, FL   32887-4800

ADVANCES IN NURSING SCIENCE
Aspen Publishers, Inc.
7201 McKinney Circle
Frederick, MO   21701

AORN Journal
National Association of Operating Room Nurses, Inc.
10170 East Mississippi Ave.
Denver, COL   80231

BIRTH
Issues in Perinatal Care and Education
Blackwell Scientific Publications
Three Cambridge Center, Suite 208
Cambridge, MA 02142

CANCER NURSING
Raven Press Ltd.
1185 Avenue of the Americas
New York, NY 10036

CRITICAL CARE NURSE
P.O. Box 611
Holmes, PA   19043

CRITICAL CARE QUARTERLY
Aspen Systems Corporation
1600 Research Blvd.
Rockville, MD 20850

GASTROENTEROLGY NURSING
Williams and Wilkins
428 East Preston St.
Baltimore, MD 21202

GERONTOLOGICAL NURSING
6900 Grove Road
Thorofare, NJ 08086

DERMATOLOGY NURSING
Anthony J. Jannetti, Inc.
North Woodbury Road
Box 56
Pitman, NJ 08071

HEART AND LUNG
The Journal of Critical Care
11830 Westline Industrial Drive
St Louis, MO   63146-3318

HOLISTIC NURSING
Aspen Publishers, Inc.
7201 McKinney Circle
Frederick, MD   21701

HOSPITALS
American Hospital Assn.
Suite 700
211 East Chicago Ave.
Chicago, IL   60611

IMAGE
Sigma Theta Tau National Society of Nursing
P.O. Box 1926
Indianapolis, IN   46206-1926

IMPRINT
National Student Nurses Assn.
555 W. 57th St.
New York, NY   10019

JOURNAL OF ET NURSING
11830 Westline Industrial Dr.
St Louis, MO   63146-3318

JOURNAL OF PEDIATRIC NURSING:
Nursing Care of Children and Families
6277 Sea Harbor Dr.
Orlando, FL 32887-4800

Manuscripts:
Cecily Betz, PhD, RN
300 UCLA Medical Plaza, Suite 3308
Los Angeles, CA   90024-6969

JOGN NURSING
Journal of Obstetric, Gynecologic, and Neonatal Nursing
Nurses Assn. of American College of Obstetricians and
Gynecologists
Downsville Pike, Route 3
Box 20-B
Hagerstown, MD 21740

JOURNAL OF STAFF DEVELOPMENT
12107 Insurance Way
Hagerstown, MD   21740

JOURNAL OF CHRISTIAN NURSING
Nurses Christian Fellowship
5206 Main St.
Downer's Grove, IL 60515-4634

JOURNAL OF THE AMERICAN DIETETIC ASSN.
216 W. Jackson Blvd., Suite 800
Chicago, IL   60606-6995

JOURNAL OF CONTINUING EDUCATION IN NURSING
Charles B. Slack Inc.
6900 Grove Road
Thorofare, NJ   08086

JOURNAL OF SCHOOL HEALTH
American School Health Assn.
7263 State Rt. 43
Kent, OH   44240

Subcriptions:
ASHA National Office
P.O. Box 708
Kent, OH   44240-0708

MCN: AMERICAN JOURNAL OF MATERNAL CHILD NURSING
Manuscripts:
555 W. 57th St.
New York, NY   10019-2961

Subscriptions:
Box 1727
Riverton, NJ 08077-7327

JOURNAL OF NURSING EDUCATION
Charles B. Slack Inc.
6900 Grove Road
Thorofare, NJ 08086

NURSE ANESTHESIA
25 Van Zant St.
E Norwalk, CT   06855

Subcriptions:
P.O. Box 3000 Dept. NA
Denville, NJ   07834

NURSE EDUCATOR
P.O. Box 1600
Hagerstown, MD 21741-1600

NURSING OUTLOOK
Editorials:
555 W. 57th St.
New York, NY 10019-2961

Subscriptions:
P.O. Box 1729
Riverton, NJ 08077-7329

NURSE PRACTITIONER
Vernon Publications
3000 Northrup Way, Suite 200
Box 96043
Bellevue, WA 98009

NURSING ADMINISTRATION
100 Insurance Way, Suite 114
Hagertown, MD   21740

NURSING ADMINISTRATION QUARTERLY
7201 McKinney Circle
Frederick, MD   21701

NURSING DIAGNOSIS
P.O. Box 801360
Santa Clarita, CA   91380-1360

Subscriptions:
JB Lippincott Co.
P.O. Box 1600
Hagerstown, MD   21741-9932

NURSING FORUM
1211 Locust Street
Philadelphia, PA   19107

NURSING MANAGEMENT
103 N. Second St., Suite 200
Dundee, IL 60118

NURSING 93
1111 Bethlehem Pike
P.O. Box 908
Springhouse, PA 19477

NURSING RESEARCH
Publications:
S-N University of Pennsylvania
420 Service Dr.
Philadelphia, PA 19104

Subscriptions:
N-Re Sub Dept.
P.O. Box 1728
Riverton, NJ 08077-7328

NURSING TIMES
Airfreight International Ltd. Inc.
2323 Randolph Ave.
Avenel, NJ 07001

NUTRITION TODAY
Manuscripts:
Helen Guthrie, PhD
S-126 Henderson Human Development Bldg.
University Park, PA 16802

Subscriptions:
Williams and Wilkins
428 E. Preston St.
Baltimore, MD 21202

ONCOLOGY NURSING FORUM
501 Holiday Drive
Pittsburgh, PA 15220-2749

PEDIATRIC NURSING
National Assn. of Pediatric Nurse
Associates and Practitioners
Anthony J. Jannetti, Inc.
North Woodbury Rd.
Box 56
Pitman, NJ 08071

RN
Medical Economics Co.
680 Kinderkamack Road
Oradell, NJ 07646

Subscription:
Box 182194
Columbus, Ohio 43272

PSYCHOSOCIAL NURSING
6900 Grove Road
Thorofare, NJ 08086

INDEX